MW01224993

Practicing Freedom: The Yoga Sutra of Patañjali

Also by Witold Fitz-Simon from Dedo Press:

Yoga Practice Journal

Practicing Freedom
The Yoga Sutra of Patañjali

Witold Fitz-Simon

A New Rendering
and Study Guide to the Ancient Classic

dedo press
New York, NY

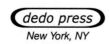

Cover Painting by Barbara Hulanicki

Published by Dedo Press
New York, NY
www.dedopress.com

Published 2006

10 9 8 7 6 5 4 3 2 1

Printed in the United States of America

ISBN: 0-9771733-1-3

to my teachers:

Fitz
Barbara
Colleen
Katchie
Robin

Contents

Introduction

The Royal Path

We know next to nothing about Patañjali, the author of the Yoga Sutra. Tradition tells us he is an incarnation of the serpent-god Ananta who descended from heaven to teach yoga to the world and is often represented in traditional statuary as a serpent, or as having a hood of many serpent heads. Many texts have been attributed to men of the name Patañjali, most significantly an exposition on Sanskrit grammar and a treatise on medicine, both of which are also ascribed to the author of the Yoga Sutra in Indian tradition. Scholars date these texts as having come from widely different periods of history, however, with the Yoga Sutra thought to be the latest of them. This means Patañjali would have to have lived for several hundred years to have written all three.

Scholarly opinion dates the Yoga Sutra as being from the second century of the Christian Era. From the text we can see that Patañjali had a deep understanding of contemporary philosophy, coupled with great skill as a teacher. In his work he was able both to synthesize and add to the body of knowledge of the time. As a rule, yogis tend less to the intellectual and more to the practical side of philosophy. Their concern is to experience directly the higher states of consciousness that lead to emancipation from the continuous and eternal suffering of the material world. Patañjali seems to have combined the best of both, providing the how and the why of yogic practice. He outlines, with surprising clarity and detail for such a short work, the underlying rationale of the yogic perspective without getting lost in minutiae. More importantly, perhaps, is the attention he pays to the actual practices the seeker must work on in order to achieve the desired freedom. It is for this reason that the Yoga Sutra has survived for two thousand years and has been referred to and adapted to fit into the schemas of many other philosophical traditions of the Indian subcontinent.

The development of Yoga itself is inextricably tied to the ancient Vedic sacrificial religion, dating back some six thousand years. What we think of as yoga today most likely bears little resemblance to the yoga of Patañjali's time. In the earliest days the union of man with the divine came in the form of elaborate ritual. As time passed a substantial body of speculative work emerged as the great sages of the Vedas retreated into the forest to ponder the nature of reality. Eventually they theorized that the sacrificial rituals could be internalized in personal disciplines. A person could achieve a union with the divine through prayer, meditation and the consuming of specialized herbs enabling him to transcend material existence and rebirth.

There are three principle ways of thinking about yoga. Thought to be derived from the Sanskrit verb *"yuj"* - to yoke, to join, to fasten together – the word can be used as a general term for any form of spiritual or meditative technique or practice. By bringing the mundane and the eternal together, the practitioner is able to realize the transcendent in our impermanent world. Over the centuries this idea has been applied to many of the different belief systems that have emerged from the foundations of Vedic literature. Thus we have Buddhist yoga as well as Jain and Hindu varieties.

Over the millennia, different approaches to liberating spiritual practices have emerged. These can be thought of not as different denominations, but as different bodies of technique. There are five major categories that are still practiced today:

Bhakti Yoga – The yoga of devotion. Involves chanting, religious ceremony and ritual sacrifice.

Karma Yoga – The yoga of action. Involves surrendering the individual sense of self to a larger cause. This involves not only charitable works, but an attitude of surrender and service in everything the *yogin* does.

Jñana Yoga – The yoga of wisdom. This is a highly intellectual mode of yoga. It involves careful study and deduction to discriminate between the transient and the eternal.

Hatha Yoga – The forceful yoga. By cultivating what the ancients termed a "diamond body," the practitioner aims to effect change on both the physical and spiritual plane through the practice of postures and breath work.

Rāja Yoga – The royal yoga. Following the techniques put forth by Patañjali in the Yoga Sutra, the *yogin* achieves freedom through the application of will power in the form of meditative practices.

In writing his seminal text, Patañjali codified existing yogic philosophy and practice, adding to it his own gloss and ideas. From this emerged a whole body of philosophical literature in the form of commentaries and expositions that evolved into one of the six orthodox philosophies of Indian thought, or *darśanas*. Classical Yoga, so named to differentiate the system from the many other interpretations of yogic ideas, shares with its sister philosophy, *Sāṃkhya*, the dualist concept that the eternal and the material are forever separate and it is the realization of this that allows the *yogin* to free himself from the misery of continued rebirths. Strictly speaking, Classical Yoga does not exist as a separate entity in the present day. Its teachings have survived, but have been re-interpreted to serve the predominant monistic (all reality is one) philosophy of Vedanta and the body-centered transformative practices of *Hatha Yoga*.

The word *sutra* means "thread", and refers to the ceremonial thread that members of the priestly caste, the *brahmin*, wear. The sutra style of writing is common in the main texts of the six classical *darśanas*. The author lays down a number of terse aphorisms to convey his ideas. These sutras are often no more than strings of words that do not even make up a full sentence. This makes the text easier to memorize, useful in what is primarily an oral tradition, with the added benefit of obscuring the meaning, requiring a teacher to interpret it for the student.

A Note On The Translation

In many of the currently available English versions, translators attempt to stay close to the *sutra* style. The result is often unwieldy and difficult to read. In this rendition I have done my best to present the concepts in a readable fashion. Wherever possible I have elaborated the sentence structure to deepen the meaning, but without loading the text with too much interpretation, saving that for the following section. In both parts, as in the study guide, I have tried to present Patañjali's concepts in a linear fashion that will allow the reader to master the ideas for him or herself. There are some sections that I have elaborated more completely and some that I have glossed over. The Yoga Sutra is not something that you read once and put away. It is a text that requires continual study, that one must return to year after year. The ideas are profound and must be lived to be fully understood.

As a teacher and practitioner, I come to the material not from a scholarly perspective, but from a practical and personal one. I began this project purely for myself. I felt a need to get inside the text and think through Patañjali's meaning for myself that I could understand it better. My hope is to provide a rendition that is easy enough to read casually, but one that also carries sufficient meaning as to serve as a guide for those who wish to mine its depths. There are many excellent scholarly translations that parse and dissect Patañjali's words, putting them in philosophical and historical context, some of which are listed in the bibliography. I encourage you to seek them out if you are of a mind to learn more. Most of us are not so academically inclined, however. It is with this in mind that I offer "Practicing Freedom" up to you.

Enstasy

One final thought before we proceed with the text. Wherever possible I have tried to present easily useable English words to stand in for many of Patañjali's technical terms. The word *samādhi* presents a problem, however. It is often translated as "integration" or "ecstasy". Though not exactly incorrect, they do not embody the full meaning of the word. In his book "Yoga: Immortality and Freedom", Mircea Eliade coined the term "enstasy", from the Greek, to refer to *samādhi*. Whereas in an ecstatic state the practitioner elevates consciousness to a higher plane by going outside the body, in an "enstatic" state, higher consciousness is achieved by going within. Though the word "enstasy" is not a common word, *samādhi* is not a state that bears any resemblance to mundane life. For this reason I have chosen to use it in the text.

The Yoga Sutra of Patañjali

samādhi pāda

samādhi pāda

I.1
atha-yoga-anuśāsanam

I.2
yogaś-citta-vṛtti-nirodhaḥ

I.3
tadā draṣṭuḥ sva-rūpe'vasthānam

I.4
vṛtti-sārūpyam-itaratra

I.5
vṛttayaḥ pañcatayaḥ kliṣṭa-akliṣṭaḥ

I.6
pramāṇa-viparyaya-vikalpa-nidrā-smṛtayaḥ

I.7
pratyakṣa-anumāna-āgāmaḥ pramāṇāni

I.8
viparyayo mithyā-jñānam-atad-rūpa-pratiṣṭham

Chapter on Enstasy

I.1
Here now begins systematic instruction in techniques of meditative discipline, referred to as "Yoga."

I.2
Yoga is the process of restriction of the fluctuations of consciousness.

I.3
Then the observer can know its own true nature.

I.4
Otherwise, the observer identifies itself with the fluctuations of consciousness.

I.5
There are five kinds of fluctuation, each of which may or may not cause suffering.

I.6
They are: right perception, misconception, conceptualization, sleep and memory.

I.7
Right perception is based on direct observation, inference or tradition.

I.8
Misconception is knowledge that is incorrectly assumed to be true.

I.9
śabda-jñāna-anupātī vastu-śūnyo vikalpaḥ

I.10
abhāva-pratyaya-ālambanā-vṛttir-nidrā

I.11
anubhūta-viṣaya-asaṃpramoṣaḥ smṛtiḥ

I.12
abhyāsa-vairāgyābhāṃ tan-nirodhaḥ

I.13
tatra sthitau yatno'bhyāsaḥ

I.14
sa tu dīrgha-kāla-nairantarya-satkāra-āsevito dṛdha-bhūmiḥ

I.15
dṛṣṭa-ānuśravika-viṣaya-vitṛṣnasya vaśīkāra-saṃjña vairāgyam

I.16
tat-paraṃ puruṣa-khyāter-guṇa-vaitṛṣṅyam

I.17
vitarka-vicāra-ānanda-asmitā-rūpa-anugamāt-saṃprajñataḥ

I.18
virāma-pratyaya-abhyāsa-pūrvaḥ saṃskāra-śeṣo'nyaḥ

I.9
Conceptualization comes as a result of verbal knowledge and not direct knowledge of an object.

I.10
Sleep is a fluctuation based on the notion of absence of conscious activity.

I.11
Memory is the not letting go of, or the recollection of experiences.

I.12
Practice and dispassion are required to restrict these fluctuations of consciousness.

I.13
Practice refers to the effort of will required to achieve stability in that restricted state.

I.14
But this practice becomes firmly grounded only after it has been properly cultivated without interruption for a long time.

I.15
Dispassion is mastered when all things outside oneself, be they directly perceived with the senses or conceptually understood, no longer evoke cravings or attachments.

I.16
The highest form of this dispassion comes when even the underlying qualities of the material universe cease to evoke craving or attachment and one becomes aware of one's true self as separate from the material universe.

I.17
Reasoning, reflection, joy and a sense of one's self as a discrete individual all accompany this state of dispassionate awareness.

I.18
Those who practice the notion of cessation, or ending, may attain the next state of dispassionate awareness which consists solely of a structure of residue from prior acts in the deep memory.

I.19
bhava-pratyayo videha-prakṛti-layānām

I.20
śraddhā-vīrya-smṛti-samādhi-prajña-pūrvaka itareṣām

I.21
tīvra-saṃvegānām-āsannaḥ

I.22
mṛdu-madhya-adhimātravāt-tato'pi viśeṣaḥ

I.23
īśvara-praṇidhānād-vā

I.24
kleśa-karma-vipāka-āsayair-aparāmṛṣṭaḥ puruṣa-viśeṣa īśvaraḥ

I.25
tatra niratiśayaṃ sarva-jña-bījam

I.26
pūrveṣām-api guruḥ kālena-anavacchedāt

I.27
tasya vācakaḥ praṇavaḥ

I.28
taj-japas-tad-artha-bhāvanam

I.19
Those who, instead, practice the notion of becoming, or material existence, will cling to and be dissolved in the primordial material world and will not achieve this deeper form of dispassionate awareness.

I.20
Trust in the path, vigor, mindfulness, enstasy and discernment must all be cultivated if one is to achieve this deeper state.

I.21
The goal is near for those who practice with extreme intensity.

I.22
Thus, there will be a difference if the effort put into practice is mild, moderate or great.

I.23
Or the goal can be achieved through devotion to the ideal of the supreme self.

I.24
This supreme self is a distinct, extraordinary self untouched by inherent causes of affliction or by action and consequence and the structure of residue that these leave behind in the deep memory.

I.25
Embodied in this soul is the unsurpassed source of all knowing.

I.26
This timeless example has also been a guide to those who have come before.

I.27
It is represented by the sacred syllable "A-U-M."

I.28
Recitation of this syllable leads to becoming steeped in its meaning.

I.29
tataḥ pratyakcetanā-adhigamo'py-antarāya-abhāvaś-ca

I.30
vyādhi-styāna-saṃśaya-pramāda-ālasya-avirati-bhrānti-darśana-alabdha-bhūmikatva-anavasthitatvāni citta-vikṣepās-te'ntarāyāḥ

I.31
duḥka-daurmanasya-aṇgam-ejayatva-śvāsa-praśvāsā vikṣepa-sahabhuvaḥ

I.32
tat-pratiṣedha-artham-eka-tattva-abhyāsaḥ

I.33
maitrī-karuṇā-muditā-upekṣānām sukha-duḥkha-puṇya-apuṇya-viṣayāṇāṃ bhāvanātaś-citta-prasādanam

I.34
pracchardana-vidhāraṇābhyāṃ vā prāṇasya

I.35
viṣaya-vatī vā pravṛttir-utpannā manasaḥ sthiti-nibandhanī

I.36
viśokā vā jyotiṣmatī

I.37
vīta-rāga-viṣayaṃ vā cittam

I.38
svapna-nidrā-jñāna-ālambanaṃ vā

I.39
yathā-abhimata-dhyānād-vā

I.29
From this develops inwardly-directed awareness. Obstacles disappear.

I.30
Sickness, apathy, doubt, negligence, laziness, self-indulgence, delusion, lack of progress and instability in that progress are distractions of consciousness. These are the obstacles.

I.31
Pain, depression, unsteadiness of the body and breath are accompanying distractions.

I.32
In order to prevent these distractions, practice one of the following principles.

I.33
Consciousness settles as a result of projecting friendliness, compassion, delight and equanimity towards all things, be they joyful, sorrowful, noble or base.

I.34
Or as a result of focusing on the exhalation of the breath and the pause before the following inhalation.

I.35
Or as a result of focusing the mind steadily on the perception of the senses.

I.36
Or as a result of contemplating sorrowless and illuminating thoughts.

I.37
Or as a result of contemplating those who have conquered attachment.

I.38
Or as a result of contemplating insights drawn from sleep and dreams.

I.39
Or as a result of any form of meditative absorption, as desired.

I.40
parama-aṇu-parama-mahatva-anto'sya vaśīkāraḥ

I.41
kṣīṇa-vṛtter-abhijātasya-iva maṇer-grahītṛ-grahaṇa-grāhyeṣu tat-stha-tad-añjanatā samāpattiḥ

I.42
tatra śabda-artha-jñāna-vikalpaiḥ saṃkīrṇā savitarkā samāpattiḥ

I.43
smṛti-pariśuddhau sva-rūpa-śūnya-iva-artha-mātra-nirbhāsā nirvitarkā

I.44
etayā-eva savicārā nirvicārā ca sūkṣma-viṣayā vyākhyātā

I.45
sūkṣma-viṣayatvaṃ ca-aliṇga-prayavasānam

I.46
tā eva sabījaḥ samādhiḥ

I.47
nirvicāra-vaiśāradye'adhyātma-prasādaḥ

I.48
ṛtaṃ-bharā tatra prajñā

I.49
śruta-anumāna-prajñābhyām-anya-viṣayā viśeṣa-arthatvāt

I.40
Mastery over the mind can be achieved even as it contemplates the most minute object to objects of the greatest magnitude.

I.41
As fluctuations of consciousness diminish, consciousness itself becomes like a transparent jewel. With regards to the observer (the grasper), the act of perception (the grasping) and the perceived object (the grasped), observer and object become the same.

I.42
As long as there is conceptual knowledge based on words and their meaning, this state of consciousness is called coincidence with thought.

I.43
When the deep memory becomes purified, when it is empty of all latent impulses, the object can be perceived as it is, without distortion. This state is called coincidence beyond thought.

I.44
When subtle objects are the focus, the two states of consciousness are similarly named, as coincidence with reflection and coincidence beyond reflection.

I.45
These subtle objects lead back to the undifferentiated substance of the primordial material universe.

I.46
These four states of consciousness – coincidence with thought and beyond thought, with reflection and beyond reflection – are called enstasy with seed.

I.47
Lucidity in the state of coincidence beyond reflection is called clarity of inner being.

I.48
In this state, insight brings absolute truth.

I.49
The nature of this insight is different from that derived by tradition and inference because of its special significance.

I.50
taj-jah saṃskāro'nya-saṃskāra-pratibandhī

I.51
tasya-api nirodhe sarva-nirodhān-nirbījaḥ samādhiḥ

I.50
The residue in deep memory born from this insight obstructs all others.

I.51
When this deep residue is also restrained, it is called enstasy without seed.

sādhana pāda

sādhana pāda

II.1
tapaḥ svādhyāya-īśvara-praṇidhānāni kriyā-yogaḥ

II.2
samādhi-bhāvana-arthaḥ kleśa-tanū-karaṇa-arthaś ca

II.3
avidyā-asmitā-rāga-dveṣa-abhiniveśāḥ pañca-kleśāḥ

II.4
avidyā kṣetram-uttareṣāṃ prasupta-tanu-vicchinna-udārāṇām

II.5
anitya-aśuci-duḥkha-anātmasu nitya-śuci-sukha-ātma-khyātir-avidyā

II.6
dṛg-darśana-śaktyor-eka-ātmatā-iva-asmitā

II.7
sukha-anuśayī rāgaḥ

Chapter on Practice

II.1
Self-discipline, self-study and devotion to the ideal of the supreme self make up the path of *Kriyā Yoga* (or Yoga of Action).

II.2
Kriyā Yoga has the dual purpose of cultivating enstasy and of attenuating the inherent causes of affliction.

II.3
These five causes of affliction are misapprehension of one's true nature, the sense of one's self as a discrete individual, attachment, aversion and the drive for self-preservation.

II.4
Misapprehension of one's true nature is the underlying cause of the other causes of affliction. These can be dormant, restricted, blocked or fully active.

II.5
Misapprehension of one's true nature is the seeing of the eternal, the pure, the joyful and the true self in that which is impermanent, impure, sorrowful and not the true self.

II.6
The sense of one's self as a discrete individual is the identification of the ability to observe with the observer itself.

II.7
Attachment follows on from pleasure.

II.8
duḥkha-anuśayī dveṣaḥ

II.9
sva-rasa-vāhī viduṣo'pi tathā rūḍho'bhiniveśaḥ

II.10
te pratiprasava-heyāḥ sūkṣmāḥ

II.11
dhyāna-heyās-tad-vṛttayaḥ

II.12
kleśa-mūlaḥ karma-āśayo dṛṣṭa-adṛṣṭa-janma-vedanīyāḥ

II.13
sati mūle tad-vipāko jāty-āyur-bhogāḥ

II.14
te hlāda-paritāpa-phalāḥ puṇya-apuṇya-hetutvāt

II.15
pariṇāma-tāpa-saṃskāra-duḥkhair-guṇa-vṛtti-virodhāc-ca duḥkham-eva sarvaṃ vivekinaḥ

II.16
heyaṃ duḥkham-anāgatam

II.17
draṣṭṛ-dṛśyayoḥ saṃyogo heya-hetuḥ

II.8
Aversion follows on from pain.

II.9
The drive for self-preservation develops of its own accord and is deeply rooted in even the wisest person.

II.10
These causes of affliction are to be overcome in their subtle form by following them inwardly back to their source through the stages of enstasy.

II.11
The fluctuations of these causes must be restricted by meditative absorption.

II.12
Action and consequence leave a residue of latent impulses in deep memory. The inherent causes of affliction are the root cause of action, consequence and these latent impulses. They may be experienced in this birth or in lives to come.

II.13
Just as this root exists, so shall its fruits: birth, life and experience.

II.14
Birth, life and experience result in delight or distress according to their cause, be it noble or base.

II.15
To the observer all is sorrow, be it from the anguish of change, the sorrow caused by latent impulses in deep memory or the conflict that arises from fluctuations of the underlying qualities of nature.

II.16
Future sorrow is that which must be overcome.

II.17
The tying together of observer with observed is the cause of that which must be overcome.

II.18
prakāśa-kriyā-sthiti-śīlaṃ bhūta-indriya-ātmakaṃ bhoga-apavarga-arthaṃ dṛśyam

II.19
viśeṣa-aviśeṣa-liṅga-mātra-aliṅgani guṅa-parvāṇi

II.20
draṣṭā dṛśi-mātraḥ śuddho'pi pratyaya-nupaśyaḥ

II.21
tad-artha eva dṛśyasya-ātmā

II.22
kṛta-arthaṃ prati naṣṭam-apy-anaṣṭaṃ tad-anya-sādhāraṇatvāt

II.23
sva-svāmi-śaktyoḥ sva-rūpa-upalabdhi-hetuḥ saṃyogaḥ

II.24
tasya hetur-avidyā

II.25
tad-abhāvāt saṃyoga-abhāvo hānaṃ tad-dṛśeḥ kaivalyam

II.26
viveka-khyātir-aviplavā hāna-upāyaḥ

II.27
tasya saptadhā prānta-bhūmiḥ prajñā

II.18
That which the observer sees, namely the material world, has the qualities of luminousness, activity and inertia. It is made tangible in the elements and the senses. It has the purpose of both enjoyment and emancipation.

II.19
The underlying qualities of the universe have four levels: the distinct, the indistinct, the differentiated and the undifferentiated.

II.20
Although the observer is, in truth, pure awareness, it sees itself as being the contents of consciousness.

II.21
The observed exists only for the sake of the observer.

II.22
Although the observed has ceased to exist for one whose purpose has been fulfilled, nevertheless, it has not ceased for others for whom it is a common experience.

II.23
It is in the bringing together of the owner and the owned that the essential nature of each is known.

II.24
The cause of this juxtaposition is misapprehension of one's true nature.

II.25
When this misapprehension disappears, the juxtaposition disappears. This cessation is pure, emancipated awareness.

II.26
The way to achieve this cessation is uninterrupted discriminating discernment between the observer and the observed.

II.27
For one who has achieved this emancipated awareness, wisdom at this last stage is sevenfold.

II.28
yoga-aṅga-anuṣṭhānād aśuddhi-kṣaye jñāna-dīptir-ā-viveka-khyāteḥ

II.29
yama-niyama-āsana-prāṇāyāma-pratyāhāra-dhāraṇā-dhyāna-samādhayo'ṣṭāv-aṅgāni

II.30
ahiṃsā-satya-asteya-brahmacarya-aparigrahā yama

II.31
jāti-deśa-kāla-samaya-anavacchinnāḥ sarva-bhaumā mahā-vratam

II.32
śauca-saṃtoṣa-tapaḥ-svādhyāya-īśvara-praṇidhānāni niyamāḥ

II.33
vitarka-bādhane pratipakṣa-bhāvanam

II.34
vitarkā hiṃsā-ādayaḥ kṛta-kārita-anumoditā lobha-krodha-moha-pūrvakā mṛdu-madhya-adhimātrā duḥkha-ajñāna-ananta-phalā iti pratipakṣa-bhāvanam

II.35
ahiṃsā-pratiṣthāyāṃ tat-saṃnidhau vaira-tyāgaḥ

II.36
satya-pratiṣṭhāyāṃ kriyā-phala-āśrayatvam

II.37
asteya-pratiṣṭhāyāṃ sarva-ratna-upasthānam

II.28
By performance of the limbs of yoga and with the dwindling of impurities, wisdom radiates up to the level of discriminating discernment.

II.29
The eight limbs of yoga are restraint, observance, posture, restraint of life-force, sense withdrawal, concentration, meditative absorption and enstasy.

II.30
The restraints are non-harming, truthfulness, non-stealing, continence and non-greed.

II.31
These are universal and apply regardless of birth, place, time or circumstance and are the great vow of yoga.

II.32
Purity, contentment, austere discipline, self-study and devotion to the ideal of the supreme self are the observances.

II.33
In order to repel unwholesome thoughts, the yogin should cultivate their opposites.

II.34
These unwholesome thoughts, such as harming and the like, whether engaged in oneself, caused to be committed or approved of in others, whether arising from greed, anger or infatuation, whether modest, medium or excessive, endlessly bear fruit in misapprehension of one's true nature and in sorrow. Thus the cultivation of their opposites.

II.35
Enmity is abandoned in the presence of one who is grounded in non-harming.

II.36
Action and consequence are rooted in truth for one who is grounded in truthfulness.

II.37
All abundance appears for one grounded in non-stealing.

II.38
brahmacarya-pratiṣthāyāṃ vīrya-lābhaḥ

II.39
aparigraha-sthairye janma-kathaṃtā-saṃbodhaḥ

II.40
śauchāt-sva-aṅga-jugupsā parair asaṃsargaḥ

II.41
sattva-śuddhi-saumanasya-eka-agrya-indriya-jaya-ātma-darśana-yogyatvāni ca

II.42
saṃtosād anuttamaḥ sukha-lābhaḥ

II.43
kāya-indriya-siddhir-aśuddhi-kṣayāt tapasaḥ

II.44
svādhyāyād-iṣṭa-devatā-saṃprayogaḥ

II.45
samādhi-siddhir-īśvara-praṇidhānāt

II.46
sthira-sukham-āsanam

II.47
prayatna-śaithilya-ananta-samāpattibhyām

II.48
tato dvandva-anabhighātāḥ

II.49
tasmin-sati śvāsa-praśvāsayor-gati-vicchedaḥ pranayamaḥ

II.38
Vitality is acquired by one grounded in continence.

II.39
Knowledge of the subtle causes of one's birth becomes available to one grounded in non-greed.

II.40
With purity comes detachment from the body and disinterest in contact with others.

II.41
With purity also comes serenity, gladness, single-pointed focus, mastery of the senses and the capacity for self-awareness.

II.42
Contentment brings the greatest joy.

II.43
Impurities dwindle with austere discipline. The body and the senses become refined.

II.44
Self-study establishes contact with one's chosen deity.

II.45
Devotion to the ideal of the supreme self brings the perfection of enstasy.

II.46
The posture of meditation should be steady and comfortable.

II.47
It should be effortlessly relaxed and infinitely expansive.

II.48
Then the yogin will be undisturbed by the buffeting of opposing forces.

II.49
With this comes control of the flow of inhalation and exhalation, or restraint of the life-force.

II.50
bāhya-abhyantara-stambha-vṛttir-deśa-kāla-saṃkhyābhiḥ paridṛṣṭo dīrgha-sūkṣmaḥ

II.51
bāhya-abhyantara-viṣaya-ākṣepī caturthaḥ

II.52
tataḥ kṣīyate prakāśa-āvaraṇam

II.53
dhāraṇāsu ca yogyatā manasaḥ

II.54
sva-viṣaya-asaṃprayoge cittasya sva-rūpa-anukāra indriyāṇāṃ pratyāhāraḥ

II.55
tataḥ paramā vaśyatā-indriyāṇām

II.50
Inhalation, exhalation and the pauses between can be conditioned according to area of focus, duration and number of repetitions to prolong and refine the breath.

II.51
The fourth aspect of breath transcends the pauses between inhalation and exhalation.

II.52
That which obscures inner light disappears.

II.53
The mind becomes fit for concentration.

II.54
Withdrawal of the senses is when the sense organs separate themselves from their objects and instead imitate the form of consciousness.

II.55
From this, the sense organs are subjugated.

vibhūti pāda

vibhūti pāda

III.1
deśa-bandhaś-cittasya dhāraṇā

III.2
tatra pratyaya-ekatānatā dhyānam

III.3
tad-eva-artha-mātra-nirbhāsaṃ sva-rūpa-śunya-iva samādiḥ

III.4
trayam-ekatra saṃyamaḥ

III.5
taj-jayāt prajña-ālokaḥ

III.6
tasya bhūmiṣu viniyogaḥ

III.7
trayam-antara-aṇgam pūrvebhyaḥ

III.8
tad-api bahir-aṅgam nirbījasya

Chapter on Powers

III.1
Concentration is the binding of consciousness to one place.

III.2
Meditative absorption is when all the notions that fill the mind are directed towards that one place.

III.3
Enstasy occurs when, in that state of meditative absorption, the object of focus shines forth as if devoid of form and the observer merges with the observed.

III.4
All three of these techniques – concentration, meditative absorption and enstasy – practiced together are known as constraint.

III.5
With mastery of constraint comes the light of insight.

III.6
This mastery progresses in stages.

III.7
These three limbs – concentration, meditative absorption and enstasy are inner limbs, compared to the previous five which are outer limbs.

III.8
Even so, they are outer limbs compared to the process of seedless enstasy.

III.9
vyutthāna-nirodha-saṃskārayor-abhibhava-prādur-bhāvau nirodha-kṣana-citta-anvayo nirodha-pariṇāmaḥ

III.10
tasya praśānta-vāhitā saṃskārāt

III.11
sarva-arthatā-ekāgratayoḥ kṣaya-udaya cittasya samādhi-pariṇāmaḥ

III.12
tataḥ punaḥ śānta-uditau tulya-pratyayau cittasya-ekāgratā-pariṇāmaḥ

III.13
etena bhūta-indriyeṣu dharma-lakṣaṇa-avasthā-pariṇāmā vyākhyātāḥ

III.14
śānta-udita-avyapadeśya-dharma-anupātī dharmī

III.15
krama-anyatvaṃ pariṇāma-anyatve hetuḥ

III.16
pariṇāma-traya-saṃyamād-atīta-anāgata-jñānam

III.17
śabda-artha-pratyayānām-itara-itara-adhyāsāt saṃkaras-tat-pravibhāga-saṃyamāt-sarva-bhūta-rūta-jñānam

III.9
That moment of transition when latent impulses that tend towards action and consequence have been subjugated and new impulses that promote further restriction emerge is called the restriction transformation.

III.10
This transformation is a calm and steady flow of restrictive latent impulses.

III.11
The dwindling of outward dissipation and the rise of single-pointed focus is called the integration transformation.

III.12
That moment when the quieting and the rising notions of consciousness become similar is called the single-pointedness transformation.

III.13
The elements and the senses undergo transformations of quality, of time span and of condition as a result of the passage of time.

III.14
The underlying substance of these three things goes through latent, emergent and unmanifested stages.

III.15
The sequence of progression of these three stages is the reason for the differentiation of the above-mentioned transformations.

III.16
Through constraint on these successive transformations comes knowledge of the past and future.

III.17
The object, the notion of the object and the name of the object all become confused as a result of being superimposed on each other. Constraint on the distinction between these three brings knowledge of the language of all beings.

III.18
saṃskāra-sākṣat-karaṇāt-pūrva-jāti-jñānam

III.19
pratyayasya para-citta-jñānam

III.20
na ca tat-sa-ālambanaṃ tasya-aviṣayī-bhūtatvāt

III.21
kāya-rūpa-saṃyamāt-tad-grāhya-śakti-stambhe cakṣuḥ-prakāśa-asaṃprayoge'ntardhānam

III.22
sa-upakramaṃ nir-upakramaṃ ca karma tat-saṃyamād-apara-anta-jñānam ariṣṭebhyo vā

III.23
maitry-ādiṣu balāni

III.24
baleṣu hasti-bala-ādīni

III.25
pravṛitty-āloka-nyāsāt sūkṣma-vyavahita-viprakṛṣṭa-jñānaṃ

III.26
bhuvana-jñānaṃ surye saṃyamāt

III.27
candre tārā-vyūha-jñānam

III.28
dhruve tad-gati-jñānam

III.18
Through direct observation of latent impulses comes knowledge of one's previous births.

III.19
Through direct observation of the notion of another one gains knowledge of that other's consciousness.

III.20
This, however, does not include knowledge of the underlying notions of that consciousness as they are not the object of constraint.

III.21
By practicing constraint on the body's form one becomes invisible. The ability to be perceived is suspended and the light that travels to the observer's eye is disrupted.

III.22
The consequences of action are either imminent or deferred. Both omens and constraint on these consequences reveal knowledge of the yogin's own death.

III.23
Constraint on friendliness, compassion and delight brings power.

III.24
Constraint on specific powers, such as those of an elephant, brings those powers.

III.25
Constraint on one's inner light brings knowledge of that which is subtle, hidden or distant.

III.26
Constraint on the sun brings knowledge of the universe.

III.27
Constraint on the moon brings knowledge of the positions of the stars.

III.28
Constraint on the pole star brings knowledge of the stars' movements.

III.29
nābhi-chakre kāya-vyūha-jñānam

III.30
kaṇṭha-kūpe kṣut-pipāsā-nivṛittiḥ

III.31
kūrma-nāḍyāṃ sthairyam

III.32
mūrdha-jyotiṣi siddha-darśanam

III.33
prātibhād-vā sarvam

III.34
hṛdaye citta-saṃvit

III.35
sattva-puruṣayor-atyanta-saṃkīrṇayoḥ pratyaya-aviśeṣo bhogaḥ para-arthatvāt sva-artha-saṃyamāt puruṣa-jñānam

III.36
tataḥ prātibha-śrāvaṇa-vedanā-ādarśa-āsvāda-vārtā jāyante

III.37
te samādhāv-upasargā vyutthāne siddhayaḥ

III.38
bandha-kāraṇa-śaithilyāt-pracāra-saṃvedanāc-ca cittasya para-śarīra-āveśaḥ

III.29
Constraint on the navel chakra brings knowledge of the body's organization.

III.30
Constraint on the throat chakra stops hunger and thirst.

III.31
Constraint on the "tortoise" subtle energy channel brings steadiness.

III.32
Constraint on the luminous crown chakra brings visions of those who are perfected.

III.33
Or all becomes known through a spontaneous flash of illumination.

III.34
Constraint on the heart brings understanding of the nature of consciousness.

III.35
Experience is caused by the lack of distinction between the true self and the luminous serenity of the material world. The material world exists for the sake of the true self, whereas the true self exists for its own sake. Constraint on the distinction between these two brings knowledge of the true self.

III.36
With this constraint comes spontaneous illumination through hearing, feeling, seeing, tasting and smelling.

III.37
These are obstacles to enstasy. They are achievements of ordinary awareness.

III.38
The entering of another's body can be accomplished by relaxing the causes of attachment to one's own and by understanding the working of consciousness.

III.39
udāna-jayāj-jala-paṇka-kaṇṭaka-ādiṣv-asaṅga utkrāntiś-ca

III.40
samāna-jayāj-jvalanam

III.41
śrotra-ākāśayoḥ saṃbandha-saṃyamād divyaṃ śrotam

III.42
kāya-ākāśayoḥ saṃbandha-saṃyamāl-laghu-tūla-samāpatteś-ca-ākāśa-gamanam

III.43
bahir-akalpitā vṛttir-mahā-videha tataḥ prakāśa-āvaraṇa-kṣayaḥ

III.44
sthūla-sva-rūpa sūkṣma-anvaya-arthavattva-saṃyamād-bhūta-jayaḥ

III.45
tato'ṇima-ādi-prādurbhāvaḥ kāya-saṃpat-tad-dharma-anabhighātaś-ca

III.46
rūpa-lāvaṇya-bala-vajra-saṃhananatvāni kāya-saṃpat

III.47
grahaṇa-sva-rūpa-asmitā-anvaya-arthavattva-saṃyamād-indriya-jayaḥ

III.48
tato mano-javitvaṃ vikaraṇa-bhāvaḥ pradhāna-jayaś-ca

III.39
Mastery over the rising current of life-force in the body brings the ability to levitate over such things as water, swamps and thorns.

III.40
Mastery over the balancing current of life-force in the body brings radiance of the body.

III.41
Constraint on the relationship between ear and ether brings clairaudience.

III.42
Constraint on the relationship between body and ether makes consciousness coincide with the lightness of cotton. In this way it becomes possible for the body to travel through space.

III.43
Constraint on a disembodied state of consciousness outside the body causes the veil that covers the inner light to dwindle.

III.44
Mastery over the elements is gained by constraint on their coarse and subtle aspects, on their essential nature, their interrelatedness and on their purpose.

III.45
From this come other powers, such as the ability to shrink to the size of an atom, perfection of the body and invulnerability.

III.46
This bodily perfection consists of beauty, grace, strength and diamond-like hardness.

III.47
Mastery over the sense organs comes from constraint on the act of perception itself, on the essential nature of the senses, on identification with them, on their interrelatedness and on their purpose.

III.48
With this the senses can function without aid of the sense organs, moving with the quickness of the mind, and gaining mastery over the underlying substance of nature.

III.49
sattva-puruṣa-anyatā-khyāti-mātrasya sarva-bhāva-adhiṣṭhātṛitvaṃ sarva-jñātṛtvaṃ ca

III.50
tad-vairāgyād api doṣa-bīja-kṣaye kaivalyam

III.51
sthāny-upanimantraṇe saṅga-smaya-akaraṇaṃ punar-aniṣṭa-prasaṅgāt

III.52
kṣaṇa-tat-kramayoḥ saṃyamād-viveka-jaṃ jñānam

III.53
jāti-lakṣaṇa-deśair-anyatā-anavacchedāt-tulyayos-tataḥ pratipattiḥ

III.54
tārakaṃ sarva-viṣayaṃ sarvathā-viṣayam-akramaṃ ca-iti viveka-jaṃ jñānam

III.55
sattva-puruṣayoḥ śuddhi-sāmye kaivalyam-iti

III.49
Discernment between the true self and the luminous serenity of the material world brings omniscience and supremacy over all states of existence.

III.50
With dispassion for even this, the seeds of imperfection dwindle and pure, emancipated awareness is achieved.

III.51
Even under the attention of celestial beings, the yogin should not smile proudly nor give cause for attachment, lest undesirable inclinations should recur.

III.52
Constraint on the fundamental unit of time and its sequence of progression brings the wisdom of discriminative discernment.

III.53
With this it becomes possible to distinguish between similar things normally indistinguishable by type, appearance or position.

III.54
The wisdom of discriminative discernment encompasses all things and transcends time and its progression.

III.55
When the mind achieves qualities of serenity and tranquility equal to the purity of the true self it has achieved pure, emancipated awareness.

kaivalya pāda

kaivalya pāda

IV.1
janma-oṣadhi-mantra-tapaḥ-samādhi-jāḥ siddayaḥ

IV.2
jāty-antara-pariṇāmaḥ prakṛty-āpūrāt

IV.3
nimittam-aprayojakaṃ prakṛtīnāṃ varaṇa-bhedas-tu tataḥ kṣetrikavat

IV.4
nirmāṇa-cittāny-asmitā-mātrāt

IV.5
pravṛtti-bhede prayojakaṃ cittam-ekam anekeṣām

IV.6
tatra dhyāna-jam anāśayam

Chapter on Freedom

IV.1
The extraordinary accomplishments are inherent in one's birth, or are achieved through the use of herbs, the recitation of mantras or through austere disciplines.

IV.2
The transformation of one thing into another comes about as a result of the abundant flow of the primordial substance of the material world.

IV.3
The underlying cause of these transformations has no aim or motive, but causes obstacles to be removed just as a farmer removes obstacles in the way of the water that irrigates his fields.

IV.4
The construct of individual consciousness comes from the underlying universal principle of sense of self as a discrete entity.

IV.5
Even though individual consciousnesses may appear to be independent, that individuality and independence originates in the underlying universal sense of the discrete self.

IV.6
Those consciousnesses that are born of meditative absorption are without latent impulses.

IV.7
karma-aśukla-akṛṣṇaṃ yoginas-trividham-itareṣām

IV.8
tatas-tad-vipāka-anuguṇānām-eva-abhivyaktir-vāsanām

IV.9
jāti-deśa-kāla-vyavahitānām-apy-āntantaryaṃ smṛti-saṃskārayor-eka-rūpatvat

IV.10
tāsām-anāditvaṃ ca-āśiso nityatvāt

IV.11
hetu-fala-āśraya-ālambanaiḥ saṃgṛahītatvād-eṣām-abhāve tad-abhāvaḥ

IV.12
atīta-anāgataṃ sva-rūpato'sty-adhva-bhedād-dharmāṇām

IV.13
te vyakta-sūkṣmā guṇa-ātmānaḥ

IV.14
pariṇāma-ekatvād-vastu-tattvam

IV.15
vastu-sāmye citta-bhedāt-tayor-vibhaktaḥ panthāḥ

IV.16
na ca-eka-citta-tantraṃ vastu tad-apramāṇakaṃ tadā kiṃ syāt

IV.7
The actions of the yogin have neither positive nor negative consequence, whereas those of others are threefold: positive, negative and of mixed consequence.

IV.8
The consequences of the latent impulses that these three kinds of action leave behind will come to fruition when conditions are favorable.

IV.9
Even though the consequence of a latent impulse may be separated from the creation of the memory that caused it by class of existence, place or time, latent impulse and memory are of the same nature. Thus there is a direct cause and effect relationship between the two.

IV.10
These latent impulses are without beginning because the universal will to manifest is eternal.

IV.11
As latent impulses are held together by cause, effect, foundation and dependence, with the negation of these, the impulses themselves shall disappear.

IV.12
Past and future exist in the changing qualities of form.

IV.13
These changing qualities of form are either manifest or subtle and are of the underling essential qualities of material existence.

IV.14
The perceived reality of an object comes from the consistency of transformation of the underlying qualities of nature.

IV.15
Given that many consciousnesses will observe the same object, consciousness and object are each of a different order.

IV.16
The existence of a given object is not dependent on being observed by any single consciousness. An unobserved object

IV.17
tad-uparāga-apekṣitvāc-cittasya vastu jñāta-ajñātam

IV.18
sadā jñātās-citta-vṛttayas-tat-prabhoḥ puruṣasya-apariṇāmitvāt

IV.19
na tat-sva-ābhāsaṃ dṛśyatvāt

IV.20
eka-samaye ca-ubhaya-anavadhāraṇam

IV.21
citta-antara-dṛśye buddhi-buddher-atiprasaṅgaḥ smṛti-saṃkaraś-ca

IV.22
citer-apratisaṃkramāyās-tad-ākāra-āpattau sva-buddhi-saṃvedanam

IV.23
draṣṭṛ-dṛśya-uparaktaṃ cittaṃ sarva-artham

IV.24
tad-asaṃkhyeya-vāsanābhiś-citram-api para-arthaṃ saṃhatya-kāritvāt

IV.25
viśeṣa-darśina ātma-bhāva-bhāvanā-vinivṛttiḥ

would be unquantifiable. What might this supposed object be?

IV.17
An object is known or not according to the coloration of consciousness that it calls forth.

IV.18
The fluctuations of consciousness are always known by their sovereign, the true self, because of its changelessness.

IV.19
Consciousness cannot be self-aware because it is, itself, a material object.

IV.20
The stuff of consciousness cannot be aware of itself and another object simultaneously.

IV.21
If, within a single being, there were another consciousness to be aware of the first, this would suppose an endless succession of consciousnesses which would cause confusion of memory.

IV.22
The true self's awareness is unchanging. Consciousness only becomes self-aware when it approximates the form of the true self.

IV.23
When consciousness is colored by both the observer and the observed, then it can know all things.

IV.24
Although consciousness is speckled with countless latent impulses, because it can only work in conjunction with another, the true self, it exists for the sake of the supreme good.

IV.25
For one who sees the distinction between consciousness and true self, the misconception that consciousness is self comes to an end.

IV.26
tadā viveka-nimnaṃ kaivalya-prāgbhāraṃ cittam

IV.27
tac-chidreṣu pratyaya-antarāṅi saṃskārebhyaḥ

IV.28
hānam-eṣāṃ kleśavad-uktam

IV.29
prasaṃkhyāne'py-akusīdasya sarvathā viveka-khyāter dharma-meghaḥ samādhiḥ

IV.30
tataḥ kleśa-karma-nivṛttiḥ

IV.31
tadā sarva-āvaraṇa-mala-apetasya jñānasya-ānantyāj-jñeyam-alpam

IV.32
tataḥ kṛta-arthānāṃ pariṇāma-krama-samāptir guṇānām

IV.33
kṣaṇa-pratiyogī pariṇāma-apara-anta-nirgrāhyaḥ kramaḥ

IV.34
puruṣa-artha-śūnyānāṃ guṇānāṃ pratiprasavaḥ kaivalyaṃ sva-rūpa-pratiṣṭhā vā citi-śaktir-iti

IV.26
Then the discerning consciousness is drawn towards absolute emancipation.

IV.27
During this progression, new distracting notions may arise as a result of latent impulses.

IV.28
These may be stilled by the same techniques described for dealing with the inherent causes of affliction.

IV.29
One who remains disinterested even in this exalted state as a result of discerning insight achieves the form of enstasy known as the "Cloud of Virtue."

IV.30
Then all causes of affliction and all consequences of action cease.

IV.31
Then all impure impediments to wisdom cease. Because of the infinite scope of this wisdom there is very little still to be known.

IV.32
Then the underlying qualities of the material universe cease their progressive and evolving transformations because their purpose has been fulfilled.

IV.33
The fundamental unit of time and the individual transformations in sequence of progression of the underlying qualities share a dependent existence. When that progression is ended both can be seen for what they are.

IV.34
Now devoid of purpose, the underlying qualities of nature flow back to their source and awareness becomes firmly established in the power of its own purity in a state of absolute emancipation.

Concepts Explained

Spirit and Matter

Puruṣa (p<u>oo</u>-roo-sha)

In amongst all the technical definitions and practical techniques that Patañjali provides us as he outlines his philosophy in the Yoga Sutra comes one succinct and rather moving passage where he states the fundamental problem and purpose of his teachings:

> *II.15*
> *To the observer all is sorrow, be it from the anguish of change, the sorrow caused by latent impulses in deep memory or the conflict that arises from fluctuations of the underlying qualities of nature.*
> *II.16*
> *Future sorrow is that which must be overcome.*
> *II.17*
> *The tying together of observer with observed is the cause of that which must be overcome.*

As you read through the Yoga Sutra, you will come across the idea of duality over and over again: the subject and the object; the seer and the seen; that which is in control and that which is subservient; that which is concrete and that which is, simply, 'other'. Unlike Vedanta, the school of philosophy that dominates Indian thought in the present day in which all of reality is ultimately one undifferentiated emanation of the divine cosmos, Patañjali's model of reality is radically dualist. There is *puruṣa* and there is *prakṛti*, and although one may color the other, the two are essentially and eternally separate. In the broadest possible terms, terms which are themselves so colored by deeply-rooted Western associations that they can only be used as a general starting point, *puruṣa* can be thought of as spirit and *prakṛti* as matter.

Patañjali himself does not provide us with a simple definition of the word *puruṣa*, possibly because the meaning he intends is in keeping with the meaning generally understood by philosophers of the time. (This is not always the case with his technical definitions, as we shall see shortly with the concept of *īśvara*.) *Puruṣa*, in Classical Yoga can be thought of as that part of us that transcends the world of material phenomena, that part of us that even transcends death. We may think we are our conscious mind, our thoughts and our notion of autobiographical identity, but in fact these are all products of nature or matter. Certainly a more subtle and refined form of matter than perhaps our bodies or the ground under our feet, but the same stuff nonetheless. Even the most unencumbered and serene manifestation of consciousness, the most enlightened of minds, is a form of gross matter. *Puruṣa*, in contrast, is the underlying self-awareness behind that. Without its influence we would be unaware automata. And yet it is wholly and completely other.

Let us look at some of these concepts in context:

I.16

The highest form of this dispassion comes when even the underlying qualities of the material universe cease to evoke craving or attachment and one becomes aware of one's true self (puruṣa) *as separate from the material universe.*

I.24

This supreme self is a distinct, extraordinary self (puruṣa) *untouched by inherent causes of affliction or by action and consequence and the structure of residue that these leave behind in the deep memory.*

III.35

Experience is caused by the lack of distinction between the true self (puruṣa) *and the luminous serenity of the material world. The material world exists for the sake of the true self, whereas the true self exists for its own sake. Constraint on the distinction between these two brings knowledge of the true self.*

III.49

Discernment between the true self (puruṣa) *and the luminous serenity of the material world brings omniscience and supremacy over all states of existence.*

III.55

When the mind achieves qualities of serenity and tranquility equal to the purity of the true self (puruṣa) *it has achieved pure, emancipated awareness.*

Puruṣa as *draṣṭṛ* (drash-tri) – "one who sees"

I.3

Then the observer (draṣṭṛ) *can know its own true nature.*

II.17

The tying together of observer (draṣṭṛ) *with observed is the cause of that which must be overcome.*

II.20

Although the observer (draṣṭṛ) *is, in truth, pure awareness, it sees itself as being the contents of consciousness.*

IV.23

When consciousness is colored by both the observer (draṣṭṛ) *and the observed, then it can know all things.*

Puruṣa as *svāmin* (swah-min) – "owner, proprietor, master or lord"

II.23

It is in the bringing together of the owner (svāmin) *and the owned that the essential nature of each is known.*

Puruṣa as *grahītṛ* (gra-hee-tri) – "one who seizes or grasps"

I.41

As fluctuations of consciousness diminish, consciousness itself becomes like a transparent jewel. With regards to the observer (grahītṛ: the grasper), *the act of perception* (the grasping) *and the perceived object* (the grasped), *observer and object coincide.*

Puruṣa as *prabhu* (prab-hoo) – "one who is superior to or more powerful than"

IV.18

The fluctuations of consciousness are always known by their sovereign (prabhu), *the true self, because of its changelessness.*

Puruṣa as *para* (pa-ra) – "other than or different from"

IV.24

Although consciousness is speckled with countless latent

impulses, because it can only work in conjunction with another (para), *the true self, it exists for the sake of the supreme good.*

The concept of *puruṣa* is very hard to grasp in its entirety. This is the heart of the experiential and practical Classical Yoga system, unlike its sister philosophy *Sāṃkhya*, which is more intellectual and theoretical. Patañjali outlines many different techniques by which the aspirant can purify his or her awareness and experience *puruṣa* directly, thus radically shifting the aspirant's center of identity from the ever-changing material world to the changeless and eternal state of pure awareness.

Let us try a thought experiment that may help us get a taste of what that pure awareness might be:

- Adjust yourself in your seat so that your posture is comfortable and steady, with the spine erect and the head balanced.
- Soften your gaze so that you become more aware of what lies in the periphery of your vision than of the words on the page.
- Become aware of the sounds flooding into your hearing. Instead of focusing on any one sound, allow them all to wash over you.
- Imagine a free-flowing, mindful state of awareness such as this, held continuously and effortlessly.
- Now strip away any recognition of the objects in your field of vision or the sounds within earshot as if you were seeing and hearing everything for the very first time.
- Strip away any recognition of meaning of the words on the page, as if the alphabet were suddenly to change into something completely unrecognizable to you.
- Furthermore, strip away any notion that what you see before you is even language. Even strip away the notion of language itself.

- Strip away any notion you might have of your own identity: your history, your thoughts, your feelings, your reactions to the world around you.
- Leave yourself with only the notion of awareness itself, not even allowing for the things of which you are aware.

If you were to achieve this state, it would only be the first in many stages of the withdrawal of consciousness from the material world towards understanding of the true nature of things. To be ultimately free of the confusion of the true self for the contents of our conscious minds requires properly cultivated and firmly grounded, uninterrupted practice over an extended period of time.

Īśvara (eesh-va-ra)

The two classical systems of thought, *Sāṃkhya* and Yoga, stand out against the Vedic philosophical traditions of India. Often lumped together in the epic literature of the region, they share many ideas which are at odds with the Vedic sacrificial religion and the other *darśanas*, or orthodox schools of thought. There are several areas which Patañjali fails to elaborate in the same depth as the *Sāṃkhya* system. In many of these it is often reasonable to turn to the exhaustively rigorous categories of existence enumerated in *Sāṃkhya* to shed light where Patañjali has chosen not to illuminate. Patañjali's idea of *īśvara*, however, is absent entirely in *Sāṃkhya* and is so different from its usage in the prevailing Vedic thought that he takes the time to explicitly define his meaning. In the Vedic sacrificial religion, *īśvara* is another term for God. *Īśvara* is the Supreme Being, the ultimate manifestation of the Divine. Patañjali keeps the concept and uses it in a similarly exalted position, though in his philosophy it has a very different, non-theistic flavor.

I.23

Or the goal can be achieved through devotion to the ideal of the supreme self (īśvara).

I.24

This supreme self (īśvara) *is a distinct, extraordinary self untouched by inherent causes of affliction or by action and consequence and the structure of residue that these leave behind in the deep memory.*

I.25

Embodied in this soul is the unsurpassed source of all knowing.

I.26

This timeless example has also been a guide to those who have come before.

I.27

It is represented by the sacred syllable "A-U-M" (praṇava).

This completely unsullied and uncompromised *puruṣa* has never been colored by matter, has never become confused and mistaken itself for that which it beholds.

"A-U-M," or its more common condensation "om," is the primary and oldest mantra in the Vedic religious tradition. Referred to in Sanskrit as *praṇava* ('humming'), this sacred syllable has been written about and expounded upon extensively in the literature of many different traditions. In each of these it is thought to represent the absolute, transcendent and eternal reality, regardless of how that is defined in any given tradition. As we can see in the text above, Patañjali ascribes it to *īśvara* in particular, rather than to *puruṣa* in general, and presents its recitation as a method of meditative focus:

I.28

Recitation of this syllable leads to becoming steeped in its meaning.

I.29

From this develops inwardly-directed awareness. Obstacles disappear.

It is possible to impose a more devotional, conventionally theistic reading onto these passages. This is, in fact, how contemporary Vedanta is able to shoehorn Patañjali into its teachings. If you take the Vedanta reading as given, however – in which all matter, all consciousness is of the same stuff, and that stuff is itself God – the flavor of this passage, along with the three later references to *īśvara*, is radically different:

II.1
Self-discipline, self-study and devotion to the ideal of the supreme self (īśvarapranidhana) *make up the path of Kriyā Yoga (or Yoga of Action).*

II.32
Purity, contentment, austere discipline, self-study and devotion to the ideal of the supreme self (īśvarapranidhana) *are the observances.*

II.45
Devotion to the ideal of the supreme self (īśvarapranidhana) *brings the perfection of enstasy.*

Devotion in this instance can then allow for the intensely ecstatic practices of Bhakti Yoga, which are diametrically opposed in methodology and purpose to Patañjali's supremely controlled and inwardly-direct techniques. This is not to suggest that Patañjali's Classical Yoga is atheistic. He does make reference to the idea of a 'chosen deity' or *iṣṭadevatā* (eesh-ta-dey-va-t<u>a</u>h):

II.44
Self-study establishes contact with one's chosen deity (iṣṭadevatā).

He has something of a negative view of celestial beings in general, however. To him they are a distraction from the path that are best ignored:

III.51
Even under the attention of celestial beings, the yogin should not smile proudly nor give cause for attachment, lest undesirable inclinations should recur.

Prakṛti (pra̲-kri-ti)

If awareness is 'other', what exactly is the 'this' that we mistake ourselves to be? Patañjali provides us with some very strong qualifiers for the material, phenomenal universe which he names *prakṛti*:

- It is impermanent, impure and sorrowful. *(II.5)*
- It has the qualities of luminousness, activity and inertia. *(II.18)*
- It is made tangible in the elements and the senses. *(II.18)*
- It has the purpose of both enjoyment and emancipation. *(II.18)*
- It exists only for the sake of the observer, the true self. *(II.21 and III.35)*
- Its substance flows abundantly. *(IV.2)*
- This flow is progressive and evolving. *(IV.32)*
- Its substance has four levels: the distinct, the indistinct, the differentiated and the undifferentiated. *(II.19)*

Let us consider the idea of substance in general and the substance of reality in particular. Patañjali's model of the material universe – this realm that we think we know intimately, in which objects have form and presence, in which events happen with cause and effect, which we observe and to which we react in a seemingly continuous stream of consciousness – goes beyond that which is empirically observable down to a level of great subtlety in much the same way as the modern scientific view of matter.

According to nuclear physics, all the matter around us is

made up of minuscule particles, known as molecules, which in turn are made up of atoms. At one point, atoms were thought to be the smallest indivisible particle of a substance. The notion of an atom is an idea that predates modern science by many generations both in the East and the West. Eventually, however, science discovered that what we thought of as atoms were not indivisible, but were in fact made up of smaller particles such as electrons, protons and neutrons. (See Figure 1.) These in turn were found to be made up of numerous other, even smaller particles. The smaller the particles the less concrete they become.

We think of an object as having some form of boundary. We think of objects as being something separate to energy. When you start to get down to the smaller, more fundamental levels of material reality, however, these distinctions begin to break down. Electrons, for example, are talked about as if they were as concrete and well-defined as, say, a river pebble. This is not strictly a falsehood, because they do exhibit properties comparable to our mundane idea of an object. An

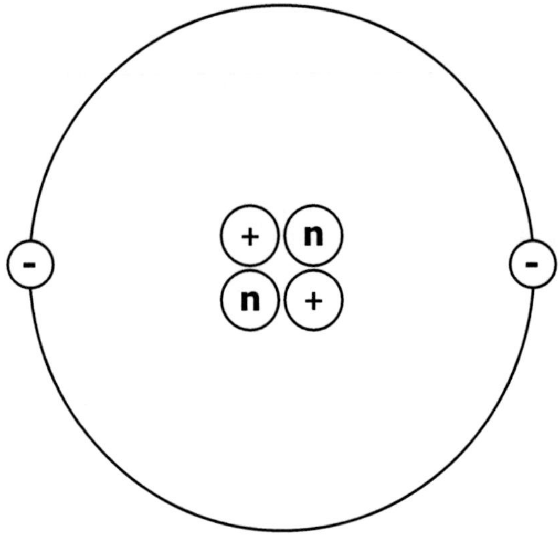

Figure 1: Schematic representation of the helium atom showing two electrons (-) orbiting around a nucleus of two protons (+) and two neutrons (n).

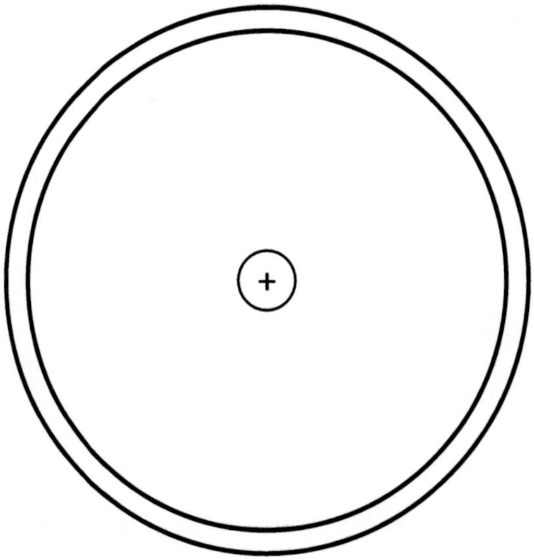

Figure 2: Representation of the hydrogen atom showing one electron shell (☰) around a nucleus of one proton (+).

electron, however, does not have a precise position around its nucleus in the same way that the moon has a precise position at any given moment around the earth. It has a range of potentialities of where it could be and around which it flows. (See Figure 2.) Think of light. As a natural phenomenon, we think of it as energy and the metaphor of a wave is used. The energy of light is transferred in much in the same way that kinetic energy, the energy of motion, is transferred by ocean waves or by sound waves through the air. It also shows properties of a particle, a discrete object. (See Figure 3.)

So which is it? Is light a wave or a particle? In a sense it is neither. It is something that exhibits the properties of both, but which we can only observe as one or the other. As you go deeper to more and more fundamental levels, the distinctions become more and more subtle, until finally you get to the level described by string theory in which all matter is made up of vibrating loops of energy strings that exist in twelve dimensions, compared to the mere three in which we exist.

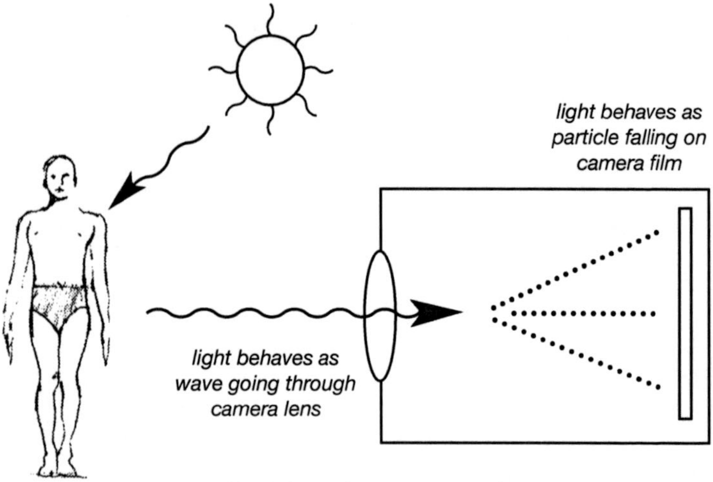

Figure 3: Particle and wave properties of light

Patañjali's model is equally deep and equally subtle, though perhaps not as elaborate as the twenty-four different categories of existence enumerated by the *Sāṃkhya* tradition. (See Figure 4.) This is in keeping with the essentially practical nature of Patañjali's philosophy. The twenty-four categories may be there, but naming and conceptualizing each of them individually does not help the yogin along the path to emancipation from the impermanent and impure sorrow of the material world. In fact, as we shall see later, any and all forms of conceptualization must ultimately be abandoned. (See sutras I.2 to I.12) So Patañjali limits himself to three fundamental qualities and to four levels of subtlety.

Guṇa (goo-na)

The philosophers of Ancient Greece theorized four archetypal elements as the fundament of the cosmos and of which all things partake: Earth, Air, Fire and Water. The idea of the elements exists in the classical philosophy of India, though there are five instead of four, as we shall see later. In the Indian cosmos, and more importantly

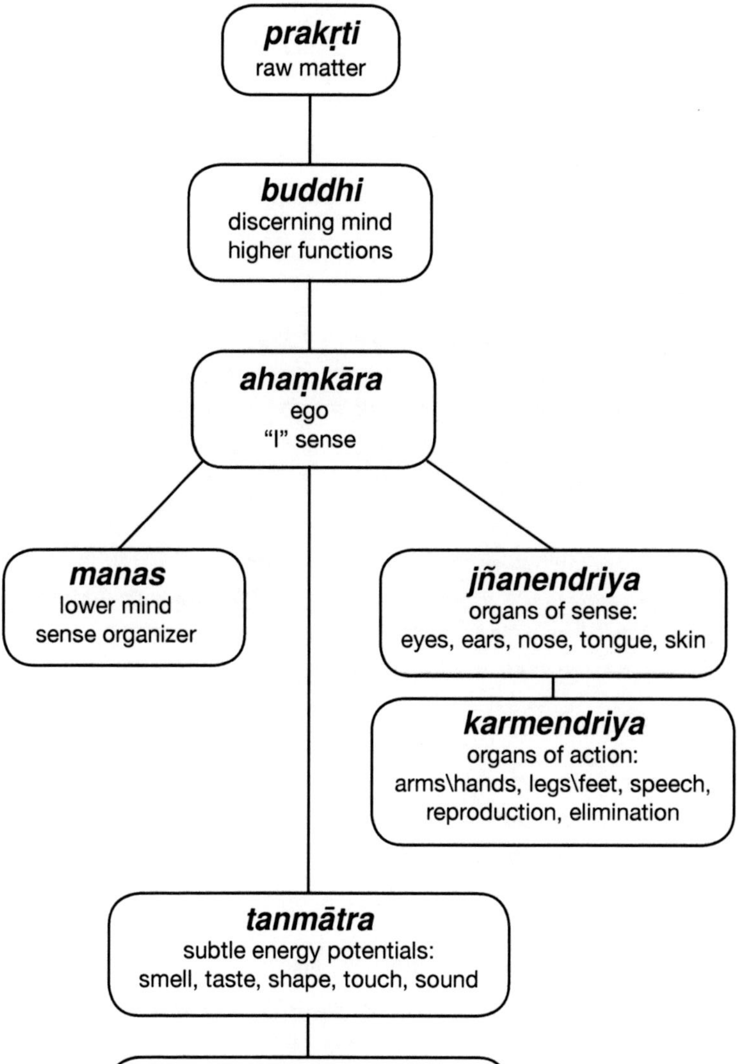

Figure 4: The twenty-four principles according to *Sāṃkhya*

for us, in the structure of reality employed by *Sāṃkhya* and Classical Yoga the elements, or *bhūta*, are in fact less subtle emanations of three even deeper fundamental substances. These three substances, known as the *guṇas*, at their most subtle level of manifestation are the material substance that makes up *prakṛti*. Though the *guṇas* have actual substance, at their root level of greatest subtlety they can be thought of as qualities or tendencies:

> *II.18*
> *That which the observer sees, namely the material world, has the qualities of luminousness* (prakāśa)*, activity* (kriyā) *and inertia* (sthiti)*. It is made tangible in the elements and the senses. It has the purpose of both enjoyment and emancipation.*

It is the tensions caused by fluctuations of the three *guṇas* that cause the unmanifested potential of *prakṛti* to become manifest in increasingly less subtle forms. The visible material world around us is its grossest, coarsest and most troubling manifestation.

> *II.15*
> *To the observer all is sorrow, be it from the anguish of change, the sorrow caused by latent impulses in deep memory or the conflict that arises from fluctuations of the underlying qualities of nature* (guṇa).

Patañjali only names the first of the above-mentioned qualities. The quality of luminousness and serenity is called *sattva*. For names of the other two, we must look to *Sāṃkhya*. The quality of activity is known as *rajas*, the quality of inertia as *tamas*. Of the three, *sattva* is the most refined. On its own, it is the part of *prakṛti* that has the potential to most resemble *puruṣa*:

> *III.55*
> *When the mind achieves qualities of serenity and tranquility*

(sattva) *equal to the purity of the true self* (puruṣa) *it has achieved pure, emancipated awareness.*

That similarity, however, leads to the fundamental confusion of *prakṛti* for *puruṣa* that underlies the problem of our sorrowful existence:

III.35
Experience is caused by the lack of distinction between the true self and the luminous serenity of the material world (sattva). *The material world exists for the sake of the true self, whereas the true self exists for its own sake. Constraint on the distinction between these two brings knowledge of the true self.*

At the most subtle and undifferentiated level of *prakṛti*, *rajas* can be thought of as the tendency to change. This would be change itself, with no underlying essence of being, no state of being from which to change nor a state of being that would be the result of that change. *Tamas* can be thought of as the principle of lack of change, but without a state of being that is failing to change. *Sattva*, in contrast, is the state of pure being with neither the tendency to change nor the tendency to stay the same. Each of these principles on their own are almost meaningless in concrete terms, as you can see by the need to define each according to concepts of the other two: being, state and change. It is the tension, conflict and fluctuation between these three principles that creates the phenomenal material world.

As consciousness and its contents are seen to be part of *prakṛti*, the *guṇas* can apply to the mind as much as to the body and the material world. *Sattva* is the source of serenity, luminousness, lightness of both body and mind. *Rajas* is the dynamic principle and is the source of all things energetic and changing. *Tamas* is the static principle, the source of all things heavy, slow and unchanging. It is easy to apply value judgments to these qualities, with *tamas* often coming out the worse for wear in our aggressive, forward-moving society. If you consider all aspects of these qualities all three can have positive and negative effects. *Rajas* can lead to mania and over-exertion as much as to positive change. *Tamas* can lead to contentment as much as to apathy and sloth. S*attva*, in turn, can lead to over-indulgence as much as to self-realization. Similarly, it is important not to think that, in the practices of Classical Yoga, one is attempting to somehow cancel out *rajas* with *tamas* or vice versa. The transformations that take place on the road to ending the underlying confusion may take place in the potentially giddy and ecstatic realm of *sattva*, but ultimately one is attempting to shift one's sense of self beyond *prakṛti* and the *guṇas* entirely. (See Figure 5.)

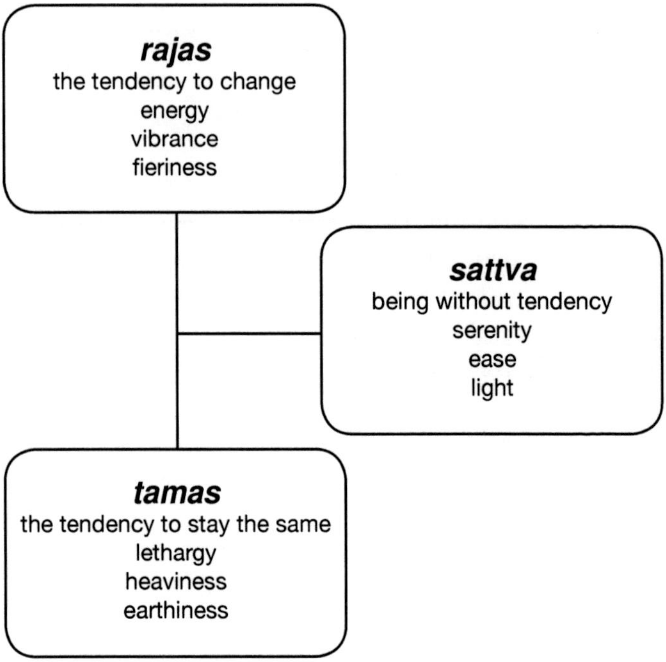

Figure 5: The three *guṇas*.

I.18

Those who practice the notion of cessation (virāma), *or ending, may attain the next state of dispassionate awareness which consists solely of a structure of residue from prior acts in the deep memory.*

I.19

Those who, instead, practice the notion of becoming (bhava), *or material existence, will cling to and be dissolved in the primordial material world* (prakṛti) *and will not achieve this deeper form of dispassionate awareness.*

These two sutras express, once again, Patañjali's dualist philosophy and offer a warning. Though he acknowledges the underlying unity of all material objects and phenomena, he makes it clear that if one operates under a non-dualist assumption that the material and divine are one and the same, all one will achieve is dissolution in *prakṛti* without even achieving the dispassionate awareness that is necessary to resolve the tensions between the three *guṇas*. One will, essentially, be derailed before one has scarcely begun.

Parvan (pa̲r-van)

II.19

The underlying qualities of the universe (guṇa) *have four levels: the distinct* (viśeṣa), *the indistinct* (aviśeṣa), *the differentiated* (liṅga-mātra) *and the undifferentiated* (aliṅga).

The first of the four levels of complexity in the stages of manifestation of the *guṇas* is referred to as *aliṅga*, or undifferentiated. The word *aliṅga* can also mean 'without sign'. At this stage, *prakṛti* and its constituent *guṇas* are nothing more than potential. They do not even exist in any concrete sense. They only achieve existence in the second stage, *liṅga-mātra*, where existence is their only characteristic. It is not until the third stage, *aviśeṣa*, that differentiation from mere existence into form takes place, though even here there is no concrete existence. Merely the underlying causes and potentials of the perceivable world and of consciousness are present. In this third stage, or *parvan*, a curious effect that Patañjali calls *asmitā-mātra* takes place.

IV.4

The construct of individual consciousness (nirmāṇa-citta) *comes from the underlying universal principle of sense of self as a discrete entity* (asmitā-mātra).

Asmitā-mātra is the first separation of subject and object, of seer and seen. In a model of reality that hinges on the distinction between awareness itself and that which is being perceived, this is the beginning of material creation. It is the first awakening of consciousness in the material realm. Something conscious will then necessitate something of which to be conscious. At this stage, awareness is still impersonal. There is no identity, no autobiography, no history. Even the idea of some form of Divine awareness does not fit here. *Asmitā-mātra* prefigures the Biblical idea of Creation exemplified in the book of Genesis: "In the beginning was the word…" It is a general notion of self that will then fragment into a myriad of individualized consciousness, or *nirmāṇa-citta*.

How, then, do you get from a "universal principle of sense of self" to the material world? On this point Patañjali is unclear, giving us only an indirect explanation:

II.18

That which the observer sees, namely the material world, has the qualities of luminousness, activity and inertia. It is made tangible in the elements (bhūta) *and the senses* (indriya). *It has the purpose of both enjoyment and emancipation.*

Something happens as a result of the generic individuation of *asmitā-mātra* that leads, in the next *parvan*, to the concrete material world. For a clue as to what this intermediary stage might be we turn to the *Sāṃkhya* system for clarification. In *Sāṃkhya*, the stage that prefigures the manifest world is called *tanmātra*, or subtle sense potential. The *tanmātras* are precursors to the five elements, or *bhūtas*. They are smell, taste, shape, touch and sound. They are, in fact, the underlying energy of all smell, taste, shape, touch and sound. We are dealing with, after all, the indistinct level of existence. From these potentials emerge, in the next, distinct *(viśeṣa)* level the five *bhūtas*: earth, air, fire and water, along with the additional element of space. (The element of space refers to the actual dimensions of an object or the amount of space an object takes up.)

This final *parvan*, *viśeṣa*, can be thought of as the surface level of *prakṛti*. On the 'object side' we have the five elements, and on the 'subject' side we have the mind. We will look at the contents of consciousness in considerable depth in a moment, but in the Yoga Sutra Patañjali makes a distinction between consciousness and mind. He uses the term *manas* (m<u>a</u>-nas) to denote that part of consciousness that organizes and manages the senses *(indriya)*. Consider these sutras in which *manas* is used and translated as 'mind':

> *I.33*
> *Consciousness* (citta) *settles...*
> *I.35*
> *...as a result of focusing the mind* (manas) *steadily on the perception of the senses.*
>
> *II.53*
> *The mind* (manas) *becomes fit for concentration.*
>
> *III.48*
> *With this the senses can function without aid of the sense organs, moving with the quickness of the mind* (manas), *and gaining mastery over the underlying substance of nature.*

As for the indriyas (sense organs), the classically held opinion, which originates in the *Sāṃkhya* tradition, is that they are ten in number. (Or possibly eleven, if you include *manas* itself.) There are five *jñanendriya* (jnya̲-nen-dri-ya), the sense organs as we would think of them: eyes, ears, nose, tongue and skin. There are also five *karmendriya* (ka̲r-men-dri-ya), or organs of action. These are the hands/arms, the feet/legs, the organs of speech, of elimination and of reproduction.

All of this breaks down into the following schema:

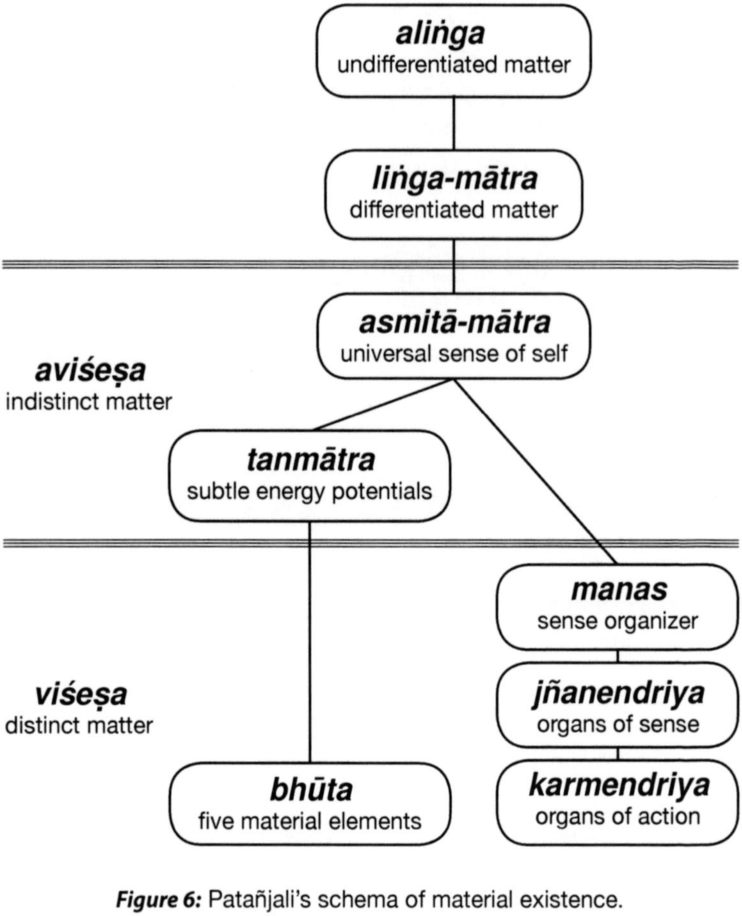

Figure 6: Patañjali's schema of material existence.

Time, Progression and Transformation

Kṣaṇa (ksha̲-na), *Krama* (kra̲-ma), and *Parināma* (pa-ri-na̲-ma)

In the very last sutra, Patañjali describes the final step in the journey of self-liberation:

> *IV.34*
>
> *Now devoid of purpose, the underlying qualities of nature* (guṇa) *flow back to their source and consciousness becomes firmly established in the power of its own purity in a state of absolute emancipation.*

The outward flow of Patañjali's four-level schema of evolution is only half the story. Just as the unmanifest, undifferentiated *(aliṅga) guṇas* flow 'outwards' to a state of concrete and distinct manifestation *(viśeṣa)*, so do they also flow back 'inwards' to their unmanifest state in a process of involution, or *pratiprasava*. If you think of *aliṅga-parvan*, the unmanifest stage, as being the bud of a flower and *viśeṣa-parvan* as being the flower in full bloom, it is as if the flower were continually blooming and regressing back into a bud, over and over again. To think of this continuous process of evolution and involution in another way, let us use the analogy of the light bulb. An electric light bulb is basically a metal wire contained in a vacuum. When connected to a circuit of alternating current, the electrical energy flows continually back and forth between the two ends of the wire. This excites the wire's component molecules so much that they heat up and glow brightly enough to illuminate a room. This is why regular light bulbs are called 'incandescent' bulbs. In a similar way, the continual sequential progression from subtle to gross, *aliṅga* to *viśeṣa*, and back again is what creates the dynamic world around us. It is this sequential progression that Patañjali calls *krama*, and upon which much of his philosophy and techniques of liberation depend.

In each cycle of evolution and involution the proportions of the three *guṇas* fluctuate, both in general terms and within each perceived object, including the contents of consciousness. The time it takes to complete one cycle of evolution and involution is, for Patañjali, the smallest unit of time, which he refers to as *kṣana*, or a 'moment':

IV.33
The fundamental unit of time (kṣana) *and the individual stages in sequence of progression* (krama) *of the underlying qualities share a dependent existence. When that progression is ended both can be seen for what they are.*

III.9
That moment (kṣana) *of transition when latent impulses that tend towards action and consequence have been subjugated and new impulses that promote further restriction emerge is called the restriction transformation* (nirodha-pariṇāma).

III.52
Constraint on the fundamental unit of time (kṣana) *and its*

sequence of progression (krama) *brings the wisdom of discriminative discernment.*

Past, present and future, as perceived by the observer, are a result of the transformations *(pariṇāma)* that occur with each cycle of *krama* and each passing *kṣana*:

IV.12
Past and future exist in the changing qualities of form.
IV.13
These changing qualities of form are either manifest or subtle and are of the underling essential qualities of material existence (guṇa).
IV.14
The perceived reality of an object comes from the consistency of transformation (pariṇāma) *of the underlying qualities of nature.*

Pariṇāma, transformation or change, is one of the key things that Patañjali is hoping we overcome:

II.15
To the observer all is sorrow, be it from the anguish of change (pariṇāma), *the sorrow caused by latent impulses in deep memory or the conflict that arises from fluctuations of the underlying qualities of nature* (guṇa).

Paradoxically, however, he wants us to capitalize on the fact that *pariṇāma* is not only inherent in the nature of *prakṛti*, but that it is also one of its main purposes:

IV.2
The transformation (pariṇāma) *of one thing into another comes about as a result of the abundant flow of the primordial substance of the material world* (prakṛti).

IV.3

The underlying cause of these transformations has no aim or motive, but causes obstacles to be removed just as a farmer removes obstacles in the way of the water that irrigates his fields.

II.18

That which the observer sees, namely the material world, has the qualities of luminousness, activity and inertia. It is made tangible in the elements and the senses. It has the purpose of both enjoyment and emancipation.

II.21

The observed exists only for the sake of the observer.

III.35

Experience is caused by the lack of distinction between the true self and the luminous serenity of the material world. The material world exists for the sake of the true self, whereas the true self exists for its own sake. Constraint on the distinction between these two brings knowledge of the true self.

All of the techniques and practices that Patañjali describes involve continuously countering the process of evolution with a self-initiated process of involution *(pratiprasava)* until, eventually, all the mechanisms buried within the contents of consciousness that promote the outward flow collapse:

IV.32

Then the underlying qualities of the material universe (guṇa) *cease their progressive and evolving* (krama) *transformations* (pariṇāma) *because their purpose has been fulfilled.*

The Contents of Consciousness

Citta (chi̱t-ta)

In Patañjali's model of what goes on in our heads, he makes a distinction between mind and consciousness. He ties his concept of manas to the physical body, organizing as it does the organs of sense and action as a medium of interaction with other objects in the field of *prakṛti.* Clearly this is only a fraction of our total mental activity. To denote the sum total of our inner conscious world he uses the term citta. Though he does not give us a concrete definition of the word, he lets us know of its nature in no uncertain terms in the fourth chapter.

Each of us may think we are a separate and unique entity, but that is only because of the manner in which *prakṛti* manifests itself. In the process of moving from merely existing without any specific form *(liṅga-mātra)* to something more concrete, the stuff of the universe begins to organize itself into two general categories, that which is observed and that which does the observing. It does this by creating an underlying point of perspective. Think of a scene being filmed for a movie. There are the sets and actors, there is the camera and there is the cameraman. The camera itself has no purpose without something to shoot and, in fact, it can be pointed at anything to start recording and make a film. There would be, however, no film without a camera and something for it to shoot. Many crew members may put their eye to the camera's viewfinder, but there is only one camera. *Asmitā-mātra*, the universal principle of a discrete self, is like the camera without someone looking through it. Each of us only has an individual point of view because of it:

> *IV.4*
> *The construct of individual consciousness* (nirmāṇa-citta) *comes from the underlying universal principle of sense of self as a discrete entity* (asmitā-mātra).
> *IV.5*
> *Even though individual consciousnesses* (citta) *may appear to be independent, that individuality and independence originates in the underlying universal sense of the discrete self.*

That said, even though Patañjali asserts that the material world emerges out of *asmitā-mātra*, he makes it clear that the world has its own independent existence. It wouldn't disappear if suddenly every living, sentient creature were to be wiped out:

> *IV.15*
> *Given that many consciousnesses* (citta) *will observe the same object, consciousness and object are each of a different order.*
> *IV.16*
> *The existence of a given object is not dependent on being observed by any single consciousness* (citta). *An unobserved object would be unquantifiable. What might this supposed object be?*

He then addresses the nature of self-awareness directly:

IV.19

Consciousness (citta) *cannot be self-aware because it is, itself, a material object.*

IV.20

The stuff of consciousness cannot be aware of itself and another object simultaneously.

IV.21

If, within a single being, there were another consciousness (citta) *to be aware of the first, this would suppose an endless succession of consciousnesses which would cause confusion of memory.*

IV.22

The true self's awareness is unchanging. Consciousness only becomes self-aware when it approximates the form of the true self.

What part of our minds is the seat of actual awareness? With *citta*, Patañjali makes a further distinction between consciousness and awareness. Awareness has nothing to do with our feelings, sensory or emotional, nor has it anything to do with our history, nor with the way in which we respond to or interact with the world. All of these things that make up *citta* are not a function of awareness, self-awareness or otherwise. They are merely stored data, instincts or learned responses. They certainly color our awareness and give shape to our sense of discrete identity, but they are not the source of what allows us to step back and be aware of our thoughts, of who we each are. That is a function of *puruṣa*. Self-awareness only happens in moments when our consciousness embodies the serene qualities of sattva to such a refined state that it mirrors *puruṣa* itself. That state of sattvic refinement is by no means a given. How often during the day are you fully self-aware? Are you fully self-aware when you watch TV or read a book? Or in moments of emotional intensity? Or when asleep? No. We 'lose ourselves' continually. This is a function of consciousness, it is inherent in the nature of *citta*. It becomes that which it observes (*samāpatti* — sa-mah-pat-ti), as Patañjali repeatedly brings to our attention:

I.4

Otherwise, the observer identifies itself with the fluctuations of consciousness.

I.41

As fluctuations of consciousness diminish, consciousness itself becomes like a transparent jewel. With regards to the observer (the grasper), the act of perception (the grasping) and the perceived object (the grasped), observer and object become the same (samāpatti).

II.17

The tying together of observer with observed is the cause of that which must be overcome.

II.20

Although the observer is, in truth, pure awareness, it sees itself as being the contents of consciousness.

Kleśa (kley-sha)

Patañjali identifies five inherent causes of affliction *(kleśa)*, five instinctive tendencies which drive our lives, the anguish which fills them and which propels us from one life to the next:

II.3

These five causes of affliction (kleśa) *are misapprehension of one's true nature* (avidyā), *the sense of one's self as a discrete individual* (asmitā), *attachment* (rāga), *aversion* (dveṣa) *and the drive for self-preservation* (abhiniveśa).

Of these, *avidyā* (a-vi-dyah) is perhaps the most important:

II.4

Misapprehension of one's true nature (avidyā), *is the underlying cause of the other causes of affliction. These can be dormant, restricted, blocked or fully active.*

II.5

Misapprehension of one's true nature (avidyā), *is the seeing of the eternal, the pure, the joyful and the true self in that which is impermanent, impure, sorrowful and not the true self.*

The second, *asmitā* (as-mi-tah) is the personalized version of the universal principle, *asmitā-mātra*.

II.6

The sense of one's self as a discrete individual (asmitā) *is the identification of the ability to observe with the observer itself.*

We confuse the information our senses bring us, our senses themselves and the analytical processes that give meaning and context to that which we are perceiving with awareness itself. Pure awareness is, after all, the most subtle part of Patañjali's schema. It is so subtle as to not have actual physical form. It makes sense, then, that it should be easily obscured by the essentially unsubtle contents and processes of our conscious minds.

The third and fourth causes of affliction are much less esoteric. We deal with them every day in one way or another:

II.7

Attachment (rāga) *follows on from pleasure.*

II.8

Aversion (dveṣa) *follows on from pain.*

Dveṣa (d-wey-sha) makes immediate sense as a cause of affliction. Pain is there to tell us that something is wrong and we have evolved mechanisms to steer us away from pain. *Rāga* (rah-ga) as an affliction may not be so immediately obvious, but think about pleasure that you anticipate in some way, but cannot have. That in itself is a kind of pain. On a subtler level, *rāga* can be thought of as the general principle of craving, which will constantly drive you outwards towards the impermanent world in order to be fulfilled.

The last of the five, *abhiniveśa* (ab-hi-ni-wey-sha), is inherent in change and mortality itself. It is one of the defining qualities of life. Without it, life would not have lasted beyond that first generation of single-celled organisms from which we all sprang.

> *II.9*
> *The drive for self-preservation* (abhiniveśa) *develops of its own accord and is deeply rooted in even the wisest person.*

These five causes of affliction are not always in play in one's mind at every second of the day:

> *II.4*
> *Misapprehension of one's true nature* (avidyā), *is the underlying cause of the other causes of affliction. These can be dormant, restricted, blocked or fully active.*

Even if they are dormant, however, they exist as a potential, forever encouraging the outward urge towards experience, anguish and rebirth and impeding the inward journey to emancipation. The very existence of the *kleśas* causes our next category of consciousness, which directly shape and inform every aspect of our daily lives.

Vṛtti (vrit-ti)

Patañjali's schema is built on the idea of energy, vibration and potential, all of which must be stilled or eradicated if freedom is to be achieved. He thinks of those mental processes that are closest to the surface as fluctuations, ripples or waves – *vṛtti* in Sanskrit – in the stuff of mind. He lists five of these *vṛttis*:

I.5
There are five kinds of fluctuation (vṛtti), *each of which may or may not cause suffering* (kliṣṭa/akliṣṭa).
I.6
They are: right perception (pramāṇa), *misconception* (viparyaya), *conceptualization* (vikalpa), *sleep* (nidrā), *and memory* (smṛti).

As we go through these, bear in mind two things. The first is that each of them may, at times, cause suffering, *kliṣṭa* (klish-ta), as much as they might not, *akliṣṭa* (a-klish-ta). The second thing to consider is that all of them, be they painful or not, must be stilled, must cease entirely to achieve the goals of Classical Yoga.

I.7
Right perception (pramāṇa) *is based on direct observation, inference or tradition.*

Pramāṇa (pra-mah-na) is any knowledge that you have derived that you can take for granted. You may have witnessed it for yourself, you may have made a logical deduction based on firm evidence in front of you, or you may have heard it from a reliable source. For example, you are holding a book in your hands at this moment. Your senses reliably inform you of the existence of the book. You can take the existence of the book for granted. Thus, the fluctuation that the book causes in your consciousness, the knowing of the book, would fall under *pramāṇa*. This type of knowledge might bring you pleasure or pain, or you might be wholly indifferent to it. In any case, it must cease.

I.8
Misconception (viparyaya) *is knowledge that is incorrectly*

assumed to be true.

Viparyaya (vi-par-ya-ya) allows for the fact that your senses may have been fooled, your reasoning may be faulty and for the fact that your reliable source might not be so reliable. Coming back to the example of the book, you might not have seen the book itself, but a friend might have told you about it. This friend might not have read the book and might have told you it was a science-fiction novel about the end of the world. Your friend is usually pretty reliable when it comes to books, so you assume that what he told you is true. Your knowledge of this book would then fall under *viparyaya*. Regardless, that knowledge must cease.

I.9
Conceptualization (vikalpa) *comes as a result of verbal knowledge and not direct knowledge of an object.*

Vikalpa (vi-kal-pa) involves any use of the imagination. Though conceptualization and imagination are potent tools for self-development, they must, in the end, cease.

I.10
Sleep (nidrā) *is a fluctuation based on the notion of absence of conscious activity.*

Nidrā (ni-drah) involves the notion of oblivion, of negation, of a complete extinguishing. This, too, is merely a fluctuation of consciousness that obscures pure awareness. This, too, must cease.

I.11
Memory (smṛti) *is the not letting go of, or the recollection of experiences.*

There are levels of memory, *smṛti* (smrit-ti), in Patañjali's schema. Here he refers to the general sense of recollection. We either recall past experience and use it as a yardstick with which to judge that which we observe and experience, or else we refuse to let past experiences die and, in effect, live in the past. Either way, *smṛti* obscures the truth and therefore must cease.

Patañjali also use the idea of *smṛti* in such a way that relates to the Freudian idea of the subconscious. This memory can be thought of as 'deep memory' and is a storehouse of the latent impressions and impulses, cravings and aversions that derive from action and consequence and drive us outward, away from our true selves and forward from birth to birth.

Karman *(ka̲r-man)*

The sacrificial rituals of the Vedic religion out of which Indian philosophical tradition emerges were incredibly complex affairs. The supremacy of the priestly social caste, the *brahmins*, grew out of this complexity, as they were the only ones trained from birth to be able to follow the ritual forms precisely. Word, gesture, posture, thought, even breath were all prescribed down to the minutest detail. A well-performed ritual would reap benefits for those on whose behalf it was performed, just as a poorly-performed ritual would bode ill. It was from this state of affairs that the idea of action and consequence, or *karman*, grew, expanding to the point of the commonly held belief that an action in a past life can even influence lives to come. Patañjali offers us a mechanism by which this happens.

The roots of all action and consequence lie in the *kleśas*:

> *II.12*
>
> *Action and consequence* (karman) *leave a residue* (āśaya) *of latent impulses in deep memory. The inherent causes of affliction* (kleśa) *are the root cause of action, consequence and these latent impulses. They may be experienced in this birth or in lives to come.*

Because we each have these five tendencies – to confuse our true selves for the contents of consciousness, to believe we are discrete individuals, to become attached to pleasurable experience, to be averse to unpleasant experience, to have a strong drive for self-preservation – we either initiate action, or respond to our environment in such a way that leaves an impression or residue, *āśaya* (ah-sha-ya). Only one who is fully emancipated is capable of acting in such a way that does not cause this residue, be it beneficial or harmful:

IV.7

*The actions of the yogin have neither positive (*aśukla *- 'not white') nor negative (*akṛṣṇa *- 'not black') consequence, whereas those of others are threefold: positive, negative and of mixed consequence.*

This residue takes the form of a latent impression or impulse, referred to as *saṃskāra* (sang-ska-ra).

II.15

To the observer all is sorrow, be it from the anguish of change (pariṇāma)*, the sorrow caused by latent impulses* (saṃskāra) *in deep memory or the conflict that arises from fluctuations* (vṛtti) *of the underlying qualities of nature* (guṇa).

These *saṃskāras* in turn organize themselves in groupings of subliminal traits, which Patañjali calls *vāsanās* (vah-sa-nah). These traits will then flourish again when the time is right, maybe not even in this lifetime, causing us to act:

IV.8

The consequences of the latent impulses (vāsanā) *that these three kinds of action leave behind will come to fruition when conditions are favorable.*

IV.9

Even though the consequence of a latent impulse (saṃskāra) *may be separated from the creation of the memory* (smṛti) *that caused it by class of existence, place or time, latent impulse and memory are of the same nature. Thus there is a direct cause and effect relationship between the two.*

Some of these *vāsanās* will even cause us to be reborn:

II.12
Action and consequence (karman) *leave a residue* (āśaya) *of latent impulses in deep memory. The inherent causes of affliction* (kleśa) *are the root cause of action, consequence and these latent impulses. They may be experienced in this birth or in lives to come.*
II.13
Just as this root exists, so shall its fruits: birth, life and experience (bhoga).
II.14
Birth, life and experience (bhoga) *result in delight* (puṇya) *or distress* (apuṇya) *according to their cause, be it noble or base.*

Though we are always adding to this residue, there was never a time for any of us when we were free of it. Never any state of unsullied 'innocence':

IV.10
These latent impulses are without beginning because the universal will to manifest is eternal.

Only *īśvara* has never been sullied by the confusion of subject for object, *avidyā*, by *kleśa*, by *karman* or by *bhoga*:

I.24
This supreme self (īśvara) *is a distinct, extraordinary self* (puruṣa) *untouched by inherent causes of affliction* (kleśa)

or by action and consequence (karman) *and the structure of residue* (āśaya) *that these leave behind in the deep memory.*

In essence, the cycle goes like this:

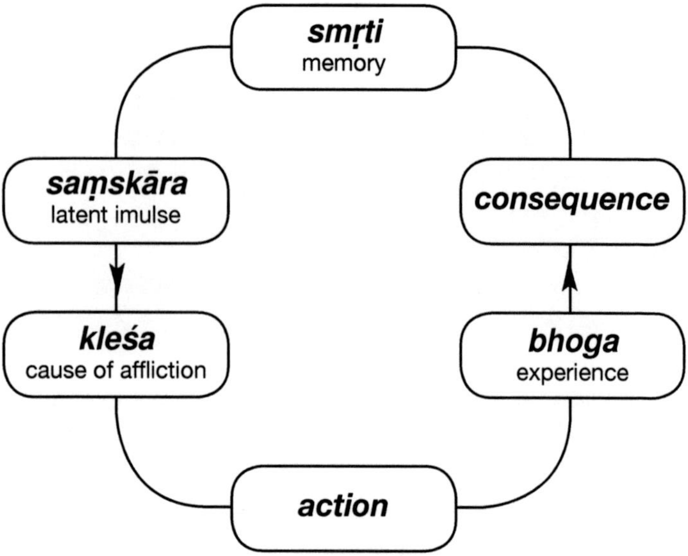

Figure 7: The *saṃskāra* cycle

Take the example of an attachment. My favorite attachment is chocolate. I have deep within me a very potent *saṃskāra* relating to the consumption of chocolate. I often find myself buying it and consuming and enjoying it often without apparent volition. This cycle would go thus:

smṛti: memories of the many times I have enjoyed the taste of chocolate.
saṃskāra: chocolate and its consumption.
kleśa: *rāga* – an attachment or craving for chocolate.
action (the first part of the *karman* continuum): I go

and buy a chocolate cookie. I eat the cookie.

bhoga: I enjoy the experience of eating the cookie, so it falls into the category of *śukla* (shu-kla) or 'white'.

consequence (the second part of the *karman* continuum): I experience delight, or *puṇya* (poong-ya).

smṛti: another pleasant memory of eating chocolate is created.

saṃskāra: the latent impulse to eat chocolate is reinforced.

The other side of the attachment/aversion dialectic might look something like this. I live on a main thoroughfare in Manhattan, with major construction on the street on a regular basis. At the peak of rush hour on a busy weekday, the combination of traffic and construction can make walking down my block very painful for the ears.

smṛti: memories of the distress and discomfort of walking down the block with major construction going on.

saṃskāra: street construction is undesirable to be around.

kleśa: *dveṣa* – an aversion to walking near street construction.

action (the first part of the *karman* continuum): I walk in the other direction and go the long way round.

bhoga: I feel relief as the noise retreats behind me, so the experience falls into the category of *śukla* or 'white'. I could just as easily have taken the shorter route, have endured the noise and the experience would have been *kṛṣṇa*, or 'black'.

consequence (the second part of the *karman* continuum): I experience delight, *puṇya*, or distress, *apuṇya* (a-poong-ya).

smṛti: either a pleasant memory of avoiding the construction is created, or an unpleasant memory of walking by it.

saṃskāra: the latent impulse to avoid street construction is reinforced.

These are both trivial examples, but they happen constantly all day long. In this way the residue, the *āśaya*, that you are born with, from previous lives and by virtue of the nature of *citta* and *prakṛti*, is continually being increased.

Let us look at a more complex example. Say you have written and recorded a song that suddenly becomes a huge success. Your face is everywhere, your name being lauded over and over, your genius as a songwriter and performer being proclaimed. This is a potentially fraught situation in terms of the activation of the *kleśas* and laying down of *saṃskāra*. This kind of attention will make you acutely aware of yourself in relation to others, fostering the idea that you are a separate individual and activating *asmitā*. The strong identification of your worth as a songwriter and performer can easily tie up that sense of identity in what you do and, in a more superficial context, in the way you look, activating *avidyā*. All that love and attention directed your way can become addictive, strongly activating the remaining three *kleśas*: *rāga* (attachment), *dveṣa* (aversion) and *abhiniveśa* (self-preservation).

I focus on a seemingly positive example, because they are the trickiest. Anyone in their right mind would want to turn away from situations that were overtly detrimental to them. An attitude of dispassion in the face of great positivity is much, much harder.

Nirodha Yoga

Nirodha (ni̱-rod-ha)

How, then, are we to begin this seemingly insurmountable process of involution, of turning back to the source? Patañjali jumps in head first, before even offering much in the way of theoretical background:

> I.2
> *yogaś-citta-vṛtti-nirodhaḥ*
> *Yoga is the process of restriction* (nirodha) *of the fluctuations* (vṛtti) *of consciousness* (citta).

This sutra is often taken as being Patañjali's definition of Classical Yoga. A process of restriction, or *nirodha*, is to happen at the various levels of absorption in the return journey back to the source, but in this sutra Patañjali is referring to restriction of the most superficial and easily accessible level of mental activity, the *vṛttis*, the fluctuations in *citta*.

If you recall, there are five *vṛttis*:

I.5

There are five kinds of fluctuation (vṛtti), *each of which may or may not cause suffering* (kliṣṭa/akliṣṭa).

I.6

They are: right perception (pramāṇa), *misconception* (viparyaya), *conceptualization* (vikalpa), *sleep* (nidrā), *and memory* (smṛti).

The yoga practice of Patañjali's day was very different to what we think of as yoga today. It was probably most comparable to seated Buddhist meditational practices. The physical postures that we practice in the average yoga class are an invention of several hundred years after his death. Though Patañjali does talk a little about posture, as we shall see later, what he refers to is a seated posture for meditation. The primary practice he advocates to achieve *nirodha* is one of single-pointed focus, or *ekāgratā* (ey-kah-gra-tah).

Abhyāsa (ab-hee-yah-sa) and *Vairāgya* (vay-rah-gya)

Before we address the actual exercises that Patañjali advocates, let us dwell a moment, as does he, on the nature of practice itself. Patañjali is very clear about what following his system entails:

I.12

Practice (abhyāsa) *and dispassion* (vairāgya) *are required to restrict* (nirodha) *these fluctuations of consciousness.*

I.13

Practice (abhyāsa) *refers to the effort of will required to achieve stability in that restricted state.*

I.14

But this practice becomes firmly grounded only after it has been properly cultivated without interruption for a long time.

"Properly cultivated without interruption for a long time." In other words, this is not an easy process, not something you can achieve on a Sunday afternoon before dinner. Though he does not put a timetable on it, he does suggest that, for some, the goal will be attainable within their present birth:

I.21
The goal is near for those who practice with extreme intensity.
I.22
Thus, there will be a difference if the effort put into practice is mild, moderate or great.

Not only must you do the exercises, but you must perform them with a particular frame of mind, that of dispassion, or *vairāgya*. Merely focusing the mind is insufficient. Powerful emotion can have that effect. How many of us have never become supremely focused in the pursuit of pleasure, or consumed with anger?

I.15
Dispassion (vairāgya) *is mastered when all things outside oneself, be they directly perceived with the senses or conceptually understood, no longer evoke cravings or attachments.*

Vairāgya is not only necessary to still the superficial mental processes, it is essential to free us from the deepest, most subtle layers of attachment:

I.16
The highest form of this dispassion comes when even the underlying qualities of the material universe (guṇa) *cease to evoke craving or attachment and one becomes aware of one's true self* (puruṣa) *as separate from the material universe.*

I.17

Reasoning, reflection, joy and a sense of one's self as a discrete individual (asmitā) *all accompany this state of dispassionate awareness.*

Interestingly enough, in the above sutra Patañjali notes that one of the *kleśas*, the inherent causes of affliction, is a result of this highest state of dispassionate awareness. Though it brings with it many positive things – reasoning, joy and reflection – it also reinforces *asmitā*, the sense of self-identity, meaning this is far from the final stage. If anything, it is merely a preparation for the real work to come. He then gives us even further caveats:

I.18

Those who practice (abhyāsa) *the notion of cessation* (virāma), *or ending, may attain the next state of dispassionate awareness which consists solely of a structure of residue from prior acts* (saṃskāra) *in the deep memory.*

I.19

Those who, instead, practice the notion of becoming (bhava), *or material existence, will cling to and be dissolved in the primordial material world and will not achieve this deeper form of dispassionate awareness.*

This is another place where Patañjali makes clear his dualist views. He tells us it is not enough to still the mind and become dispassionate. If the aspirant seeks to become one with all of material creation, that is what will happen. It is, in fact, all that will happen. He or she will become absorbed by *prakṛti* and will never achieve true emancipation. Only by working from the underlying premise that all fluctuation, all emanation from the undifferentiated source, can cease entirely to reveal the pure awareness that exists separate from it will the aspirant find true emancipation. Patañjali calls for the cultivation of devotion, either to the path itself:

I.20

Trust in the path, vigor, mindfulness, enstasy and discernment must all be cultivated if one is to achieve this deeper state.

...or to *īśvara*, the supreme self, the highest form of divinity such as it exists in Patañjali's schema:

I.23

Or the goal can be achieved through devotion to the ideal of the supreme self (īśvarapranidhana).

Antarāya (an-ta-rah-ya) and *Vikṣepa* (veek-shey-pa)

It is encouraging to know that even two thousand years ago aspirants suffered from the same obstacles, *antarāya*, and distractions, *vikṣepa*, that we do today:

I.30

Sickness, apathy, doubt, negligence, laziness, self-indulgence, delusion, lack of progress and instability in that progress are distractions (vikṣepa) *of consciousness* (citta). *These are the obstacles* (antarāya).

I.31

Pain, depression, unsteadiness of the body and breath are accompanying distractions (vikṣepa).

•

Tattva-abhyāsa (tat-va-ab-hee-yah-sa)

After this overview of what must be done and the approach in which to do it, he provides us with several concrete principles *(tattva)* of practice *(abhyāsa)*. The first is repetition of the sacred syllable, *praṇava*:

I.28
Recitation of this syllable leads to becoming steeped in its meaning.
I.29
From this develops inwardly-directed awareness. Obstacles (antarāya) *disappear.*

He groups this technique earlier in the text along with his explanation of *īśvara*. There then follows a long list of possible techniques of practice, both to overcome the obstacles and to still the mind:

I.33
Consciousness settles as a result of projecting friendliness, compassion, delight and equanimity towards all things, be they joyful, sorrowful, noble or base.

This first technique can be taken in two ways. The first is exactly as described, a general emanation of these four virtuous emotions towards all beings everywhere. The second is to apply the individual emotions towards the specific criteria listed by Patañjali. Thus one would bestow friendliness on those who are filled with joy, compassion for those who are filled with sorrow, delight towards those of virtuous and noble character and equanimity towards those with base or negative intentions.

I.34
Or as a result of focusing on the exhalation of the breath and

the pause before the following inhalation.

This could include both simple breath observation and more complicated pranayama practices.

I.35
Or as a result of focusing the mind steadily on the perception of the senses.
I.36
Or as a result of contemplating sorrowless and illuminating thoughts.
I.37
Or as a result of contemplating those who have conquered attachment.
I.38
Or as a result of contemplating insights drawn from sleep and dreams.

Patañjali then allows room for other possible meditative practices:

I.39
Or as a result of any form of meditative absorption, as desired.

Kriyā Yoga

Kriyā Yoga (kree-yah yo-ga)

Once the aspirant has mastered the first level of techniques and has achieved *nirodha* of the *vṛttis*, then one can begin to deal with the *kleśas* directly. To achieve this, Patañjali has devised the system of *Kriyā Yoga*, or the Yoga of Action.

> *II.2*
> Kriyā Yoga *has the dual purpose of cultivating enstasy and of attenuating the inherent causes of affliction* (kleśa).

There are three practices central to the practice of *KriyāYoga*:

> *II.1*
> *Self-discipline* (tapas), *self-study* (svādhyāya) *and devotion to the ideal of the supreme self* (īśvarapranidhana) *make up the path of* Kriyā Yoga *(or Yoga of Action).*

Īśvarapranidhana refers to an attitude of devotion to *īśvara*, which is to say a complete re-orienting of one's life towards the ideal of emancipation. *Svādhyāya* (swahd-hee-yah-ya) refers to intense study of the scriptures and, in modern interpretations, investigation into the nature of one's own consciousness. *Tapas* refers to any of the focusing and stilling practices that Patañjali has put forward.

II.10

These causes of affliction are to be overcome in their subtle form by following them inwardly back to their source (pratiprasava) *through the stages of enstasy.*

II.11

The fluctuations (vṛtti) *of these causes must be restricted by meditative absorption* (dhyāna).

When Patañjali use the word *vṛtti* in this case, he is not referring to the five *vṛttis* named earlier. *Vṛtti* here merely describes the energetic manner in which the *kleśas* manifest themselves. *Pratiprasava* refers to the inwardly-directed progression the aspirant undergoes through the three-fold practices of *Kriyā Yoga* and the state of meditative absorption, *dhyāna* (d-hee-yah-na), that follows on once the five *vṛttis* have been stilled. More on that later.

The reason for neutralizing and eliminating the *kleśas* is to terminate the turbulent and self-perpetuating cycle of *kleśa-karman-vipāka-āśaya* (cause of affliction-action-consequence-deposit in deep memory).

II.12

Action and consequence (karman) *leave a residue* (āśaya) *of latent impulses in deep memory. The inherent causes of affliction* (kleśa) *are the root cause of action, consequence and these latent impulses. They may be experienced in this birth or in lives to come.*

II.13

Just as this root exists, so shall its fruits: birth, life and experience (bhoga).

II.14

Birth, life and experience (bhoga) *result in delight* (puṇya) *or distress* (apuṇya) *according to their cause, be it noble or base.*

The primary concern of *Kriyā Yoga* is neutralizing and eliminating *saṃyoga* (s<u>ang</u>-yo-ga), which is the name Patañjali gives to the bringing together of observer with observed caused by *avidyā*, the source of all the other *kleśas*.

II.17

The tying together of observer with observed (saṃyoga) *is the cause of that which must be overcome.*

Fortunately, *saṃyoga* itself provides us with the opportunity to achieve emancipation, which Patañjali names *kaivalya* (k<u>ai</u>-val-ya):

II.23

It is in the bringing together (saṃyoga) *of the owner and the owned that the essential nature of each is known.*

II.24

The cause of this juxtaposition is misapprehension of one's true nature (avidyā).

II.25

When this misapprehension (saṃyoga) *disappears, the juxtaposition disappears. This cessation is pure, emancipated awareness* (kaivalya).

And how to achieve this cessation?

II.26

The way to achieve this cessation is uninterrupted discriminating discernment between the observer and the observed (viveka).

Viveka (vi-ve-ka) does not mean an intellectual understanding of what is observer and what is observed. It implies a state of profound moment-to-moment awareness and discrimination between that which is being grasped, the act of grasping itself and that which is doing the grasping, to use Patañjali's own metaphor. This would be a state in which such discernment is not optional, but is instead pivotal. This discernment needs to be so ingrained that it is perpetual, that it informs every aspect of the way you interact with the world and with your own conscious processes.

Aṣṭāṅga Yoga

Aṣṭāṅga Yoga (ash-t<u>ang</u>-ga y<u>o</u>-ga)

Kriyā Yoga, with its three limbs, is often overlooked in favor of the eight *(aṣṭa)* limbed *(aṅga)* system also outlined by Patañjali in the Yoga Sutra. Probably a quotation from earlier teachings which no longer survive in written form, *Aṣṭāṅga Yoga* details a more comprehensive approach to yogic practice that prescribes attitude and approach towards daily, mundane life as much as it does to the higher pursuit of emancipation.

> *II.28*
> *By performance of the limbs* (aṅga) *of yoga and with the dwindling of impurities, wisdom radiates up to the level of discriminating discernment* (viveka).
> *II.29*
> *The eight limbs of yoga are restraint* (yama), *observance* (niyama), *posture* (āsana), *restraint of life-force* (prāṇāyāma), *sense withdrawal* (pratyāhāra), *concentration* (dhāraṇā), *meditative absorption* (dhyāna), *and enstasy* (samādhi).

Though these eight limbs can be divided into three groups of increasing introversion - *yama* (ya-ma) and *niyama* (ni-ya-ma) dealing with the yogin's relationship and conduct with regards to the world and him or herself; *āsana* (ah-sa-na), *prāṇāyāma* (pra-na-ya-ma) and *pratyāhāra* (pra-ti-ya-ha-ra), dealing with harnessing and focusing the body, mind and senses; *dhāraṇā* (d-hah-ra-nah), *dhyāna* (d-hee-ya-na) and *samādhi* (sam-ahd-hi) representing the subtlest and innermost work – the idea is not that each of these limbs be practiced in some form of sequential order. Certainly each limb requires those previous to be effective, but each builds on the others to achieve simultaneous fulfillment in the last, *samādhi*.

The first two, *yama* and *niyama*, have five elements each and are something akin to the ten commandments for the aspiring yogin. Patañjali even refers to the *yamas* as the "Great Vow of Yoga," or *mahā-vratam* (ma-ha-vra-tam).

II.30
The restraints (yama) *are non-harming* (ahiṃsā), *truthfulness* (satya), *non-stealing* (asteya), *continence* (brahmacarya) *and non-greed* (aparigraha).
II.31
These are universal and apply regardless of birth, place, time or circumstance and are the great vow of yoga (mahāvratam).
II.32
Purity (śauca), *contentment* (saṃtoṣa), *austere discipline* (tapas), *self-study* (svādhyāya) *and devotion to the ideal of the supreme self* (īśvarapranidhana) *are the observances* (niyama).

(Note how Patañjali has singled out *tapas*, *svādhyāya* and *īśvarapranidhana* from *Aṣṭāṅga Yoga* for his *Kriyā Yoga*.)

Before going on to explain the various aspects of *yama* and *niyama*, Patañjali throws in another practical technique to aid us, cultivation of the opposite or *pratipakṣa bhāvana* (pra-ti-pak-sha b-hah-va-na).

II.33

In order to repel unwholesome thoughts, the yogin should cultivate their opposites (pratipakṣa bhāvana).

II.34

These unwholesome thoughts, such as harming and the like, whether engaged in oneself, caused to be committed or approved of in others, whether arising from greed, anger or infatuation, whether modest, medium or excessive, endlessly bear fruit in misapprehension of one's true nature and in sorrow. Thus the cultivation of their opposites (pratipakṣa bhāvana).

Following that, Patañjali goes down the list of the five *yama* - *ahiṃsā* (a-heeng-sah), *satya* (sat-ya), *asteya* (as-tey-ya), *brahmacarya* (bra-h-ma-char-ya), *aparigraha* (a-pa-ri-gra-ha) – and the five *niyama* – *śauca* (sha-oo-ca), *saṃtoṣa* (sang-to-sha), *tapas* (ta-pas), *svādhyāya* (swahd-hee-yah-ya), *īśvarapranidhana* (eesh-va-ra-pra-nid-ha-na):

II.35

Enmity is abandoned in the presence of one who is grounded in non-harming (ahiṃsā).

II.36

Action and consequence are rooted in truth for one who is grounded in truthfulness (satya).

II.37

All abundance appears for one grounded in non-stealing (asteya).

II.38

Vitality is acquired by one grounded in continence (brahmacarya).

II.39

Knowledge of the subtle causes of one's birth becomes available to one grounded in non-greed (aparigraha).

II.40

With purity (śauca) *comes detachment from the body and*

disinterest in contact with others.

II.41

With purity also comes serenity, gladness, single-pointed focus, mastery of the senses and the capacity for self-awareness.

II.42

Contentment (saṃtoṣa) *brings the greatest joy.*

II.43

Impurities dwindle with austere discipline (tapas). *The body and the senses become refined.*

II.44

Self-study (svādhyāya) *establishes contact with one's chosen deity.*

II.45

Devotion to the ideal of the supreme self (īśvarapranidhana) *brings the perfection of enstasy* (samādhi).

As mentioned before, *āsana* refers to any seated posture suitable to hold for extended periods of time for the purpose of meditation:

II.46

The posture (āsana) *of meditation should be steady and comfortable.*

II.47

It should be effortlessly relaxed and infinitely expansive.

II.48

Then the yogin will be undisturbed by the buffeting of opposing forces.

Presumably these opposing forces would be things that might affect the attempt at long periods of meditation practice, such as tension and looseness, light and dark, hot and cold, tiredness and alertness. Out of that equanimity comes a deeper awareness, which allows the yogin to manipulate the breath. In the esoteric anatomy of the Vedic tradition the underlying life force that animates all things, *prāṇā* (pra-na) is carried on the breath and can be manipulated and controlled through breath control. Thus *prāṇāyāma* is synonymous with breath control, specifically with practices that suspend the breath either retaining it in the body after the inhalation, or out of the body after exhalation. Not only does this have a subtle effect on the energies of the body, as evinced by Patañjali's reference in II.51 to a 'fourth aspect' of breath, but it stabilizes the *citta* to allow for concentration of the mind *(dhāraṇā).*

> *II.49*
> *With this comes control of the flow of inhalation and exhalation, or restraint of the life-force* (prāṇāyāma).
> *II.50*
> *Inhalation, exhalation and the pauses between can be conditioned according to area of focus, duration and number of repetitions to prolong and refine the breath.*
> *II.51*
> *The fourth aspect of breath transcends the pauses between inhalation and exhalation.*
> *II.52*
> *That which obscures inner light disappears.*
> *II.53*
> *The mind becomes fit for concentration* (dhāraṇā).

The fifth limb, *pratyāhāra*, involves more than simply closing the eyes. It requires the complete involution of the mechanisms of sensory awareness, unhinging them from the material world.

> *II.54*
> *Withdrawal of the senses* (pratyāhāra) *is when the sense organs* (indriya) *separate themselves from their objects and instead imitate the form of consciousness.*
> *II.55*
> *From this, the sense organs* (indriya) *are subjugated.*

Dhāraṇā, concentration, is a prerequisite for *dhyāna*, meditative absorption. *Dhāraṇā* is perhaps the last of the stages that one can actively practice. *Dhyāna* is something that happens of its own accord once all the preceding factors are met. When someone says they are meditating, what they are in fact doing is concentrating in a particular way towards a particular end. If they are skilled at this, then they will fall into a state of meditative absorption.

III.1
Concentration (dhāraṇā) *is the binding of consciousness to one place.*
III.2
Meditative absorption (dhyāna) *is when all the notions* (pratyaya) *that fill the mind are directed towards that one place.*

Pratyaya is another of Patañjali's technical terms that denotes a particular aspect of *citta*. More than just a *vṛtti*, it can be thought of as the cognitive representation of an object, the idea or notion of an object, or the knowledge of that object. These 'objects' can be concrete and external, or they can be more subtle, such as particular pieces of knowledge, or even concepts, specific instances of each category of *vṛttis*.

The last of the eight limbs is *samādhi*. I have used the word 'enstasy' to denote *samādhi* in English, largely because it is a technical definition and has no real equivalent in the English language. If you think of 'ecstasy' as the expansion of consciousness outward and beyond the self to achieve revelation, 'enstasy' can be thought of as the obverse. It is the going inwards to find revelation.

III.3
Enstasy (samādhi) *occurs when, in that state of meditative absorption* (dhyāna), *the object of focus shines forth as if devoid of form and the observer merges with the observed.*

In *samādhi* the observer is aware of the observed as it is without any attached notions or associations. There is only the awareness of the observer, without any interfering *avidyā*.

Samādhi and Kaivalya

Samādhi (sam-ahd-hi)

Samādhi is both a state and a process. Though it is a considerable achievement, it has many levels. It is not itself the final goal, as we shall see. Patañjali lists six different levels, each more interiorized than the last.

We have come across the idea of *samāpatti* (sa-mah-pat-ti), the quality of *citta* to become that which it observes:

> *I.41*
>
> *As fluctuations* (vṛtti) *of consciousness diminish, consciousness itself becomes like a transparent jewel. With regards to the observer (the grasper), the act of perception (the grasping) and the perceived object (the grasped), observer and object become the same* (samāpatti).

Here in the early stages of *samādhi*, Patañjali identifies four different levels of *samāpatti*: *nirvitarka-samāpatti* (coincidence with thought), *savitarka-samāpatti* (coincidence beyond thought), *nirvicāra-samāpatti* (coincidence with reflection), *savicāra-samāpatti* (coincidence beyond reflection).

I.42

As long as there is conceptual knowledge (vikalpa) *based on words and their meaning, this state of consciousness is called coincidence with thought* (nirvitarka-samāpatti).

I.43

When the deep memory (smṛti) *becomes purified, when it is empty of all latent impulses, the object can be perceived as it is, without distortion. This state is called coincidence beyond thought* (savitarka-samāpatti).

I.44

When subtle objects are the focus, the two states of consciousness are similarly named: as coincidence with reflection (nirvicāra-samāpatti) *and coincidence beyond reflection* (savicāra-samāpatti).

In the first two, *nirvitarka-samāpatti* and *savitarka-samāpatti*, the yogin's mental processes are still focusing on gross, physical objects of *viśeṣa-parvan*, the 'distinct' material world. ('*Vitarka*' means 'cogitation', or the capacity to think.) In the second two, *nirvicāra-samāpatti* and *savicāra-samāpatti*, the yogin's mental processes are focusing on subtle objects, such as the *tanmātras*, or subtle sense potentials, and even all the way back through the remaining parvans to *aliṅga-parvan*, the unmanifest and undifferentiated level of *prakṛti*.

I.45

These subtle objects lead back to the undifferentiated substance of the primordial material universe (aliṅga).

Patañjali assigns these four to the category *sabīja-samādhi*, (sa-bee-ja sam-ahd-hi) or enstasy 'with seed', meaning that they are centered on some object or other, be it subtle or gross.

I.46

These four states of consciousness – coincidence with thought and beyond thought, with reflection and beyond reflection – are called enstasy with seed (sabīja-samādhi).

In sutra I.17, Patañjali uses the word *'saṃprajñāta'* (sang-praj-nyah-ta), which means to be aware or conscious, to refer to these states of dispassionate awareness.

I.17

Reasoning (vitarka), *reflection* (vicāra), *joy* (ānanda) *and a sense of one's self as a discrete individual* (asmitā) *all accompany this state of dispassionate awareness* (saṃprajñāta).

Based on this sutra, these states are often given the name *saṃprajñāta samādhi*, or conscious enstasy, as opposed to the following stage, which he names *nirbīja-samādhi*, often referred to by commentators as *asaṃprajñāta samādhi*, seedless enstasy or enstasy beyond conscious thought:

I.47

Lucidity in the state of coincidence without reflection (nirvicāra) *is called clarity of inner being.*

I.48

In this state, insight brings absolute truth.

I.49

The nature of this insight is different from that derived by tradition and inference because of its special significance.

I.50

The residue (saṃskāra) *in deep memory born from this insight obstructs all others.*

I.51

When this deep residue is also restrained, it is called enstasy without seed (nirbīja-samādhi).

In this next stage, the process gains a certain internal momentum feeding on itself to burn out the impurities that lead outwards from the source. Patañjali denotes certain landmarks, when transformations *(pariṇāma)* occur that fundamentally alter the yogin's mental processes:

III.9
That moment of transition when latent impulses (saṃskāra) *that tend towards action and consequence have been subjugated and new impulses that promote further restriction emerge is called the restriction transformation* (nirodha-pariṇāma).
III.10
This transformation is a calm and steady flow of restrictive latent impulses (saṃskāra).
III.11
The dwindling of outward dissipation and the rise of single-pointed focus (ekāgratā) *is called the integration transformation* (samādhi-pariṇāma).
III.12
That moment when the quieting and the rising notions (pratyaya) *of consciousness* (citta) *become similar is called the single-pointedness transformation* (ekāgratā-pariṇāma).

Patañjali goes on to give us a reason for these transformations:

III.13
The elements (bhūta) *and the senses* (indriya) *undergo transformations* (pariṇāma) *of quality, of time span and of condition as a result of the passage of time.*
III.14
The underlying substance of these three things goes through latent, emergent and unmanifested stages.

III.15

The sequence of progression (krama) *of these three stages is the reason for the differentiation of the above-mentioned transformations* (pariṇāma).

At this stage, by practicing the final three stages of *Aṣṭāṅga Yoga* together and focusing them upon various objects or aspects of oneself, the yogin can gain any number of special powers, as enumerated in the third book.

III.4

All three of these techniques – concentration (dhāraṇā), *meditative absorption* (dhyāna), *and enstasy* (samādhi) *– practiced together are known as constraint* (saṃyama).

These powers, or *vibhūti* (vib-hoo-ti), gained through *saṃyama* (sang-ya-ma), can help the yogin to understand the workings of *prakṛti* better, or they can be a distraction and lead the yogin astray.

Failing that, the yogin may then progress to the final stage in the process of *samādhi*:

IV.25

For one who sees the distinction between consciousness and true self, the misconception that consciousness is self comes to an end.

IV.26

Then the discerning consciousness is drawn towards absolute emancipation (kaivalya).

Progression to the final stages is still not guaranteed, however:

IV.27

During this progression, new distracting notions (pratyaya) *may arise as a result of latent impulses* (saṃskāra).

IV.28

These may be stilled by the same techniques described for dealing with the inherent causes of affliction (kleśa).

If you recall, these techniques are self-discipline *(tapas)*, self-study *(svādhyāya)* and devotion to the ideal of the supreme self *(īśvarapranidhana)*.

IV.29

One who remains disinterested even in this exalted state as a result of discerning insight (viveka) *achieves the form of enstasy known as the "Cloud of Virtue"* (dharma-megha-samādhi).

This is the state of discernment referred to in II.26:

II.26

The way to achieve this cessation is uninterrupted discriminating discernment between the observer and the observed.

Though there is still a little way to go from *dharma-megha-samādhi*, the goal is near:

IV.30

Then all causes of affliction (kleśa) and all consequences of action (karman) *cease.*

IV.31

Then all impure impediments to wisdom cease. Because of the infinite scope of this wisdom there is very little still to be known.

IV.32

Then the underlying qualities of the material universe (guṇa) *cease their progressive and evolving* (krama) *transformations* (pariṇāma) *because their purpose has been fulfilled.*

IV.33
The fundamental unit of time (kṣaṇa) *and the individual transformations* (pariṇāma) *in the sequence of progression* (krama) *of the underlying qualities share a dependent existence. When that progression is ended both can be seen for what they are.*

Kaivalya (kai-val-ya)

Once *dharma-megha-samādhi* has become firmly established, the final changes begin to occur:

IV.34
Now devoid of purpose, the underlying qualities of nature (guṇa) *flow back to their source* (pratiprasava) *and awareness becomes firmly established in the power of its own purity in a state of absolute emancipation* (kaivalya).

This idea of the *guṇas* flowing back to their source must have presented some philosophical problems for Patañjali with the regards to the nature of objective reality. He peppers in two sutras to clarify his position:

II.22
Although the observed has ceased to exist for one whose purpose has been fulfilled, nevertheless, it has not ceased for others for whom it is a common experience.

IV.16
The existence of a given object is not dependent on being observed by any single consciousness (citta). *An unobserved object would be unquantifiable. What might this supposed object be?*

And what might this state of emancipation be like?

III.55

When the mind achieves qualities of serenity and tranquility (sattva) *equal to the purity of the true self* (puruṣa) *it has achieved pure, emancipated awareness* (kaivalya).

Serenity and tranquility devoid of suffering. Pure being without tendency to change, nor even to stay the same. No time, no transformation – the ultimate transformation having already taken place. The mechanisms that drive *citta* are completely obliterated to the point that all differentiation of matter dissolves and the stuff of mind regresses back to the primordial state of *prakṛti, aliṇga-parvan.* That means there is no fear at any level, either from simple aversion to pain or from the profound fear of one's own mortality. Similarly there is no attachment to pleasure, no anxiety and anticipation, no craving or addiction. The emancipated yogin's sense of self is not predicated on his or her former personality construct. That sense of self is completely and permanently re-centered beyond the phenomenal world to *puruṣa.* Identity and personality become meaningless at this stage, as *puruṣa* is beyond these things.

Patañjali does not say much more about *kaivalya* than the above aphorisms. It is, after all, something that can only be experienced. It cannot be described, as that would put it back in the realm of words and concepts which, by definition, it is beyond. The only other clue Patañjali gives us is in the word *'kaivalya'*, which is itself derived from *'kevala'*. *Kevala* means to be alone, to be isolated, to be completely unconnected to anything else. *Kaivalya* means the perfect completeness, the perfect aloneness of seeing. The yogin's perspective becomes one of absolute awareness, without anything to change or obscure that. It is a radical shift beyond all others from which he or she can never be diverted.

•

Appendix

Overview

Book I: Samādhi Pāda - On Enstasy

I.1 to *I.4*	Introduction and opening definitions.
I.5 to *I.11*	On the five fluctuations of consciousness.
I.12 to *I.17*	On practice and dispassion.
I.18 to *I.20*	Requirements of the path of yoga.
I.21 to *I.22*	The effects of varying intensities of practice.
I.23 to *I.26*	The supreme self.
I.27 to *I.29*	On the sacred syllable "A-U-M."
I.30 to *I.31*	On obstacles and distractions to practice.
I.32 to *I.39*	Principles of practice to avert the obstacles and distractions.
I.40	The nature of mastery over the mind.
I.41	The nature of consciousness as the fluctuations begin to settle.
I.42 to *I.46*	Definitions of higher states of consciousness and the process of "coincidence".
I.47 to *I.49*	Extrapolation of the state of lucidity in coincidence beyond reflection.
I.50	Definition of "enstasy without seed."

Book II: Sādhana Pāda - On Practice

II.1 to *II.2*	Definition and purpose of the path of *Kriyā Yoga*.
II.3 to *II.9*	Definition of the five causes of affliction.
II.10 to *II.11*	On overcoming the causes and their fluctuations.
II.12 to II.14	On the relationship between action and consequence, birth and experience.
II.15 to II.17	On the nature of sorrow.
II.18 to *II.19*	On the underlying qualities of the universe.
II.20 to *II.23*	On the relationship between observer and observed.
II.24 to *II.25*	On the misapprehension of one's true nature.
II.26 to *II.27*	On discriminating discernment and emancipated awareness.
II.28 to *II.29*	The eight limbs of yoga.
II.30 to *II.31*	The restraints.
II.32	The observances.
II.33 to *II.34*	On the repulsion of unwholesome thoughts by the cultivation of their opposites.
II.35 to *II.39*	Expansion on the nature of the restraints.
II.40 to *II.45*	Expansion on the nature of the observances.
II.46 to *II.48*	Expansion on the nature of the posture of meditation.
II.49 to *II.53*	Expansion on the nature of the restraint of life-force.
II.54 to *II.55*	Expansion on the nature of withdrawal of the senses.

Book III: Vibhūti Pāda - On Powers

III.1	Expansion on the nature of concentration.
III.2	Expansion on the nature of meditative absorption.
III.3	Expansion on the nature of enstasy.
III.4 to *III.8*	Expansion on constraint.
III.9 to *III.10*	On the restriction transformation.
III.11	On the integration transformation.
III.12	On the single-pointedness transformation.

III.13 to *III.52*	On the powers and insights gained by constraint on various phenomena.
III.53 to *III.54*	On discriminative discernment and the final stage on the yogic path.

Book IV: Kaivalya Pāda - On Freedom

IV.1	On the means to achieve the extraordinary powers.
IV.2 to *IV.3*	On obstacles and transformation.
IV.4 to *IV.6*	On consciousness and identity.
IV.7 to *IV.9*	On action, consequence, cause and effect.
IV.10 to *IV.11*	On the origin of latent impulses.
IV.12 to *IV.16*	On the nature of objective reality.
IV.17 to *IV.22*	On self-awareness.
IV.23 to *IV.24*	On the nature and purpose of consciousness.
IV.25 to *IV.26*	On the distinction between consciousness and true self.
IV.27 to *IV.28*	On dealing with distractions in the later stages.
IV.29 to *IV.33*	On the "Cloud of Virtue".
IV.34	On the final stage that leads to absolute emancipation.

•

Study Guide

Spirit and Matter

1. puruṣa (poo-roo-sha)

(See: I.16, I.24, III.35, III.49, III.55, IV.18, IV.34)

Spirit, soul, pure awareness. That part of the self that transcends the changes of the material world, that even transcends death. Not material, it can be said to have no attributes or qualifiers.

Also referred to as:

draṣṭṛ (drash-tri) – "one who sees"

(See: I.3, II.17, II.20, IV.23)

svāmin (swah-min) – "owner, proprietor, master or lord"

(See: II.23)

grahītṛ (gra-hee-tri) – "one who seizes or grasps"

(See: I.41)

prabhu (prab-hoo) – "one who is superior to or more powerful than"

(See: IV.18)

para (pa-ra) – "other than or different from"

(See: IV.24)

2. *īśvara* (<u>ee</u>sh-va-ra)
(See: I.23 to I.27)

In Classical Yoga, the closest thing to the ultimate manifestation of the Divine. A unique *puruṣa* that has never been made manifest in the material world and therefore has never been tainted by matter or the inherent causes of affliction *(kleśas)*.

praṇava (pr<u>a</u>-na-va)
(See: I.27 to I.29)

The sacred syllable "A-U-M" – or "OM" – and is represented by the character " ॐ ". It is the representation of *īśvara*. Recitation of the syllable is one of the methods Patañjali gives for gaining insight, stilling the mind and overcoming obstacles in the path of Yoga.

īśvarapranidhana (<u>ee</u>sh-va-ra-pra-nid-ha-na)
(See: II.1, II.32, II.45)

Devotion to the ideal of *īśvara*. One of the limbs of *Kriyā Yoga*, as well as one of the observances *(yama)* of *Aṣṭāṅga Yoga*.

īṣṭadevatā (eesh-ta-dey-va-t<u>ah</u>)
(See: II.44)

One's chosen deity, with whom contact can be established through self-study *(svadhyāyā)* of the scriptures.

3. *prakṛti* (pr<u>a</u>-kri-ti)
(See: IV.2, IV.3)

The primordial substance of which all things material, all things that can undergo change, are made:

- It is impermanent, impure and sorrowful. *(II.5)*
- It has the qualities of luminousness, activity and inertia. *(II.18)*

- It is made tangible in the elements and the senses. *(II.18)*
- It has the purpose of both enjoyment and emancipation. *(II.18)*
- It exists only for the sake of the observer, the true self. *(II.21 and III.35)*
- Its substance flows abundantly. *(IV.2)*
- This flow is progressive and evolving. *(IV.32)*
- Its substance has four levels: the distinct, the indistinct, the differentiated and the undifferentiated. *(II.19)*

4. guṇa (goo-na)

(See: I.16, II.15, II.18, II.19, IV.13, IV.32, IV.34)

The components of *prakṛti*. The underlying qualities of nature:

sattva (sat-va)

(See: II.41, III.35, III.49, III.55)

The quality of serenity and luminousness. *Citta*, or the contents of consciousness, most approximates *puruṣa* when its qualities become pure *sattva*.

rajas (ra-jas)

(See: II.18)

The quality of energy and change. Not referred to by name in the *Yoga Sutra*.

tamas (ta-mas)

(See: II.18)

The quality of heaviness and inertia. Also not referred to by name.

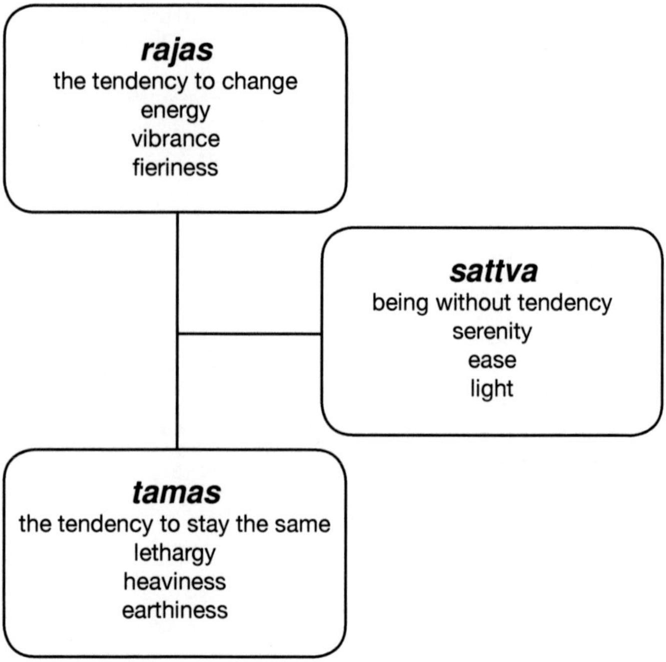

Figure 8: The three *guṇas*.

5. parvan (pa̲r-van)

(See: II.19)

The four different levels of existence:

aliṅga parvan (a̲-ling-ga pa̲r-van)

(See: I.45, II.19)

The undifferentiated level, where the constituent qualities are mere potential.

liṅga mātra parvan (li̲ng-ga ma̲h̲-tra pa̲r-van)

(See: II.19)

The differentiated level, where all it can be said of the constituent qualities is that they exist.

aviśeṣa parvan (a̲-vi-shey-sha pa̲r-van)

(See: II.19)

The indistinct level, where subject and object are first separated. The first awakening of consciousness in the aspect of an archetypal sense of self as a discrete entity.

viśeṣa parvan (vi̲-shey-sha pa̲r-van)

(See: II.19)

The distinct level, which we experience as the world around us.

asmitā mātra (as-mi-ta̲h̲ ma̲h̲-tra)

(See: IV.4)

The universal sense of self as a discrete entity, from which emerge the many individual consciousnesses.

bhūta (b-ho̲o̲-ta)

(See: II.18, III.13, III.44)

The five material elements: earth, water, air, fire and space.

manas (ma̲-nas)

(See: I.35, II.53, III.48)

The mind, specifically the part that manages and organizes the senses.

indriya (i̲n-dri-ya)

(See: II.18, II.41, II.43, II.54, II.55, III.13, III.47)

The senses.

tanmatra (ta̲n-ma-tra)

(From the Sāṃkhya system of philosophy.)

The subtle sense potentials: smell, taste, shape, touch, sound.

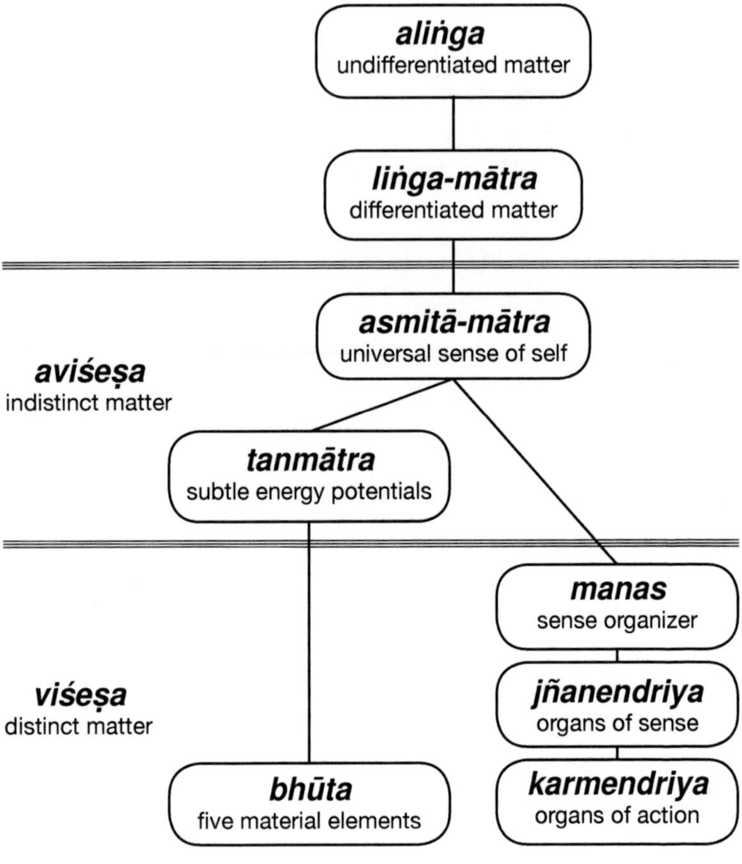

Figure 9: Patañjali's schema of material existence.

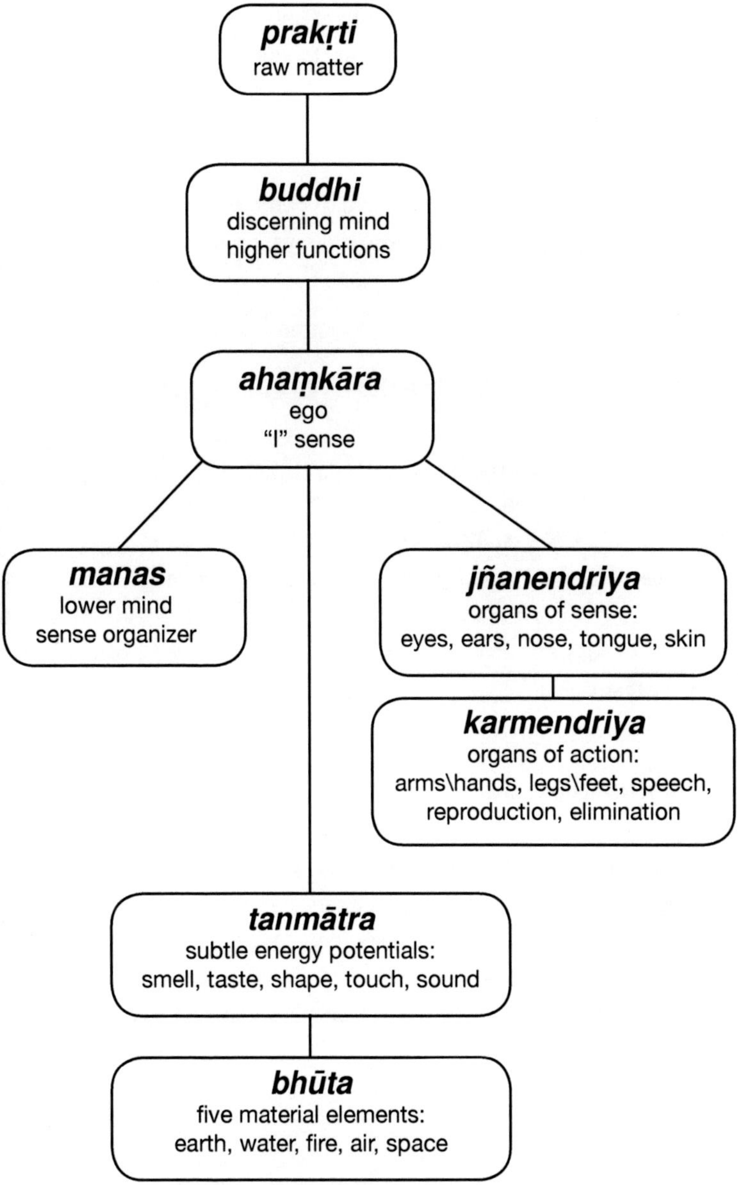

Figure 10: The twenty-four principles according to *Sāṃkhya*

jñanendriya (j-nyan-en-dri-ya)

(From the Sāṃkhya system of philosophy)

The organs of sense: eyes, ears, nose, tongue skin.

karmendriya (kar-men-dri-ya)

(From the Sāṃkhya system of philosophy)

The organs of action: arms/hands, legs/feet, organs of speech, organs of reproduction, organs of elimination.

Time, Progression and Transformation

1. kṣaṇa (ksha-na)

(See: III.9, III.52, IV.33)

The fundamental unit of time. The time it takes for *prakṛti* to flow outwards from *aliṅga* to *viśeṣa* and back to *aliṅga* again. This unit and the transformations that the *guṇas* go through are dependent on each other.

2. krama (kra-ma)

(See: III.15, III.52, IV.32, IV.33)

The sequence of the progression from one form into another as a result of the passage of time, or of the progression from *aliṅga* to *viśeṣa* and back. In the final stages of the journey described by Patañjali, once one has achieved the state of "Cloud of Virtue" or *dharma-megha-samādhi*, this progression ends and the yogin can see *kṣaṇa* and *parināma* for what they are.

3. parināma (pa-ri-na-ma)

(See: II.15, III.9, III.11 to III.13, III.15 to III.16, IV.2, IV.14, IV.32 to IV.33)

The idea of transformation. Transformation is inherent in *prakṛti*, coming as a result of it being so plentiful and flowing. In general terms it is one of the causes of sorrow and is one of the things the path of Classical Yoga aims to overcome. Perceived reality builds up because, even though everything is in a constant state of flux from undifferentiated to distinct matter and back again, the distinct form of most objects is largely consistent, giving the illusion of continuity. The sense of past, present and future emerges from a gradual shift in the consistency of form of the objects around us as they go through each successive cycle of *kṣaṇa* and *krama*.

Patañjali also names three specific transformations in the subtle progression of the contents of consciousness towards ultimate emancipation. The practice of *saṃyama* (concentration, meditation and enstasy combined) focusing on these three transformations gives the yogin the power of knowledge of past and future.

nirodha pariṇāma (ni-rod-ha pa-ri-nah-ma)

(See: III.9 to III.10)

The "restriction transformation"; when the *saṃskāras* have been subjugated and new *saṃskāras* begin to emerge that promote further restriction.

samādhi pariṇāma (sa-mahd-hi pa-ri-nah-ma)

(See: III.11)

The "integration transformation"; when the outward dissipation of *citta* begins to dwindle and a consistent state of single-pointed focus emerges.

ekāgratā pariṇāma (ey-kah-gra-tah pa-ri-nah-ma)

(See: III.12)

The "single-pointedness transformation"; when the quieting and the dissipating contents of *citta* become balanced.

The Contents of Consciousness

1. *citta* (chit-ta)

(See: I.2, I.30, I.33, I.37, II.54, III.1, III.9, III.11, III.12, III.19, III.34, III.38, IV.4, IV.5, IV.15 to IV.18, IV.21, IV.23, IV.26)

A blanket term that Patañjali uses to denote "consciousness", which is distinct from self-awareness in his schema. *Citta* cannot be self-aware because it is of *prakṛti*, and is thus a material object, albeit very subtle and refined. It cannot be aware of itself and something else simultaneously. Self-awareness only happens when the quality of *citta* (specifically, the *sattva* component) approaches the nature of *puruṣa*.

In the level of existence *(aviśeṣa-parvan)* that immediately prefigures the distinct material world *(viśeṣa-parvan)* around us, the archetypal principle of the sense of self, *(asmitā-mātra)* divides *prakṛti* into subject and object. This leads to:

nirmāṇa-citta (ni-mah-na cit-ta)

(See: IV.4, IV.5)

The construct of individual consciousness, derived from the universal principle of the sense of self as a discrete entity and reinforced by the *kleśas*, the inherent causes of affliction. Individual consciousness may appear to be independent, but this is, in fact, not the case.

2. *kleśa* (kley-sha)

(See: I.24, II.2, II.3, II.12, IV.28, IV.30)

The fundamental causes of affliction inherent in all of us. They can be dormant, restricted, blocked or fully active. They are the root cause of repeated births, of life and of experience. They are best attenuated by the practices of *Kriyā Yoga*. The five *kleśas* are:

avidyā (a-vi-dyah)

(See: II.3, II.4, II.5, II.24)

Misapprehension of one's true nature, or mistaking that which is eternal, pure and joyous, namely *puruṣa*, with that which is impermanent, impure and sorrowful, or *prakṛti*. The underlying cause of all the other causes of affliction, as well as the underlying cause of all our suffering.

asmitā (as-mi-tah)

(See: I.17, II.3, II.6, IV.4)

The sense of one's self as a discrete individual. The identifying of the ability to observe with the observer. (What might be thought of as "ego" in the Freudian and Vedanta use of the word.) A personalized version of *asmitā-mātra*, the universal principle of individuation.

rāga (rah-ga)

(See: I.37, II.3, II.7)

Attachment, which follows on from pleasure.

dveṣa (dwey-sha)

(See: II.3, II.8)

Aversion, which follows on from pain.

abhiniveśa (ab-hi-ni-wey-sha)

(See: II.3, II.9)

The drive for self-preservation. It develops of its own accord and is deeply-rooted in all of us.

3. vṛtti (vrit-ti)

(See: I.2, I.4, I.5, I.10, I.41, II.11, III.43, IV.18)

Fluctuation, ripples or waves in the stuff of consciousness. There are five of these, each of which may (*kliṣṭa* – klish-ta) or may not (*akliṣṭa* – a-klish-ta) cause suffering. Regardless of this, all of these modes of thought must be stilled if the seeker is to free him or herself of suffering. The five *vṛttis* are:

pramāṇa (pra-mah-na)

(See: I.6, I.7)

Right perception. Any knowledge that you have derived that you can comfortably take for granted, either witnessed directly, deduced logically from firm evidence, or informed of by a reliable source.

viparyaya (vi-par-ya-ya)

(See: I.6, I.8)

Misconception. Any knowledge you may have derived that turns out not to be true for whatever reason.

vikalpa (vi-kal-pa)

(See: I.6, I.9)

Conceptualization. Any use of the imagination. Conceptual knowledge based on words and their meaning.

nidrā (ni-drah)

(See: I.6, I.10)

Sleep. The idea of oblivion, negation, or complete extinguishing of awareness.

4. *karman* (ka̲r-man)

(See: I.24, II.12, III.22, IV.7, IV.30)

Colloquially referred to as *karma*, though the colloquial meaning is only half the story. Literally, *karman* means "action", but in this context, it also implies the consequences of the action. Actions can have three kinds of consequence: white (positive), black (negative) or mixed. The actions of the liberated yogin are free of all consequence, both "not-white" and "not-black".

aśukla (a̲-shu-kla)

(See: IV.7)

Not white. Without positive consequence, though without being negative in character.

akṛṣṇa (a̲-krish-na)

(See: IV.7)

Not black. Without negative consequence, though without being positive in character.

5. *āśaya* (a̲h-sha-ya)

(See: I.24, II.12)

The residue left behind in the deep memory by action and consequence, caused by the *kleśas*.

saṃskāra (sang-ska̲h-ra)

(See: I.18, I.50, II.15, III.9, III.10, III.18, IV.9, IV.10, IV.27)

The latent impressions or impulses that make up the *āśaya* laid down in the deep memory. Only *īśvara* has never been unsullied by *saṃskāra*. As for the rest of us, there was never a time, or a birth, when we were not sullied by *saṃskāra*. *Saṃskāras* are without beginning, Patañjali tells us, as the universal will to manifest is eternal.

appendix: study guide

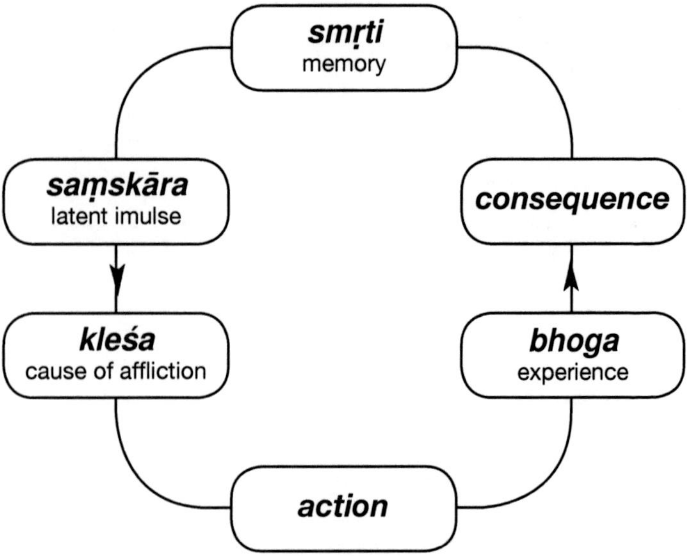

Figure 11: The *saṃskāra* cycle

vāsanā (vah-sa-nah)

(See: IV.8, IV.24)

Individual *saṃskāras* organize themselves into clusters, or *vāsanās*, of subliminal traits which flourish when conditions are most favorable, which could be in the yogin's current birth, or in births to come.

bhoga (b-ho-ga)

(See: II.13, II.18, III.35)

Used to mean both enjoyment and experience, both of which are inextricably tied to the material world and which can fall into two categories:

puṇya (poong-ya)

(See: I.33, II.14)

Auspicious, meritorious, noble, pleasant or delightful.

apuṇya (a-poong-ya)

(See: I.33, II.14)

Impure, unpleasant, wicked, base.

Nirodha Yoga

1. nirodha (ni-rod-ha)

(See: I.2, I.12, I.51, III.9)

In general, a process of restriction. Specifically, the restriction of the five *vṛttis*. The beginning of the inwardly redirecting of consciousness back to the source.

abhyāsa (ab-hee-yah-sa)

(See: I.12, I.13, I.18, I.32)

Practice. The first of the two requirements necessary for the restriction of the *vṛttis*. Patañjali defines it as "the effort of will required to achieve stability in that restricted state. But this practice becomes firmly grounded only after it has been properly cultivated without interruption for a long time."

vairāgya (vay-rah-gya)

(See: I.12, I.15, III.50)

Dispassion. The second of the two requirements necessary for the restriction of the *vṛttis*. Patañjali defines it as "when all things outside oneself, be they directly perceived with the senses or conceptually understood, no longer evoke cravings or attachments."

2. virāma (vi-rah-ma)

(See: I.18)

The idea of cessation. The requisite notion to be practiced if the yogin is to penetrate beneath the level of the *vṛttis* to the next state of dispassionate awareness.

bhava (b-h<u>a</u>-va)

(See: I.19)

The idea of becoming. A diversion from the path, practicing with this notion in mind will lead to dissipation in the material world and will prevent further penetration and ultimate freedom.

3. antarāya (an-ta-r<u>ah</u>-ya)

(See: I.30)

Obstacles on the path: sickness, apathy, doubt, negligence, laziness, self-indulgence, delusion, lack of progress and instability in that progress.

vikṣepa (v<u>ee</u>k-shey-pa)

(See: I.31)

Accompanying distractions to the obstacles: pain, depression, unsteadiness of the body and of the breath.

4. tattva-abhyāsa (tat-va ab-hee-y<u>ah</u>-sa)

(See: I.28, I.33 to I.39)

Methods of practice recommended by Patañjali for stilling the *vṛttis*:

- Recitation of "A-U-M."
- Projecting friendliness, compassion, delight and equanimity towards the joyful, the sorrowful, the noble or the base.
- Focusing on the exhalation of the breath and the pause that follows it.
- Focusing on the perception of the senses.
- Contemplating sorrowless and illuminating thoughts.
- Contemplating those who have conquered attachment.
- Contemplating insights from sleep and dreams.
- Any form of meditative absorption, as desired.

Kriyā Yoga

1. *kriyā yoga* (kri-yah yo-ga)

(See: II.1, II.2)

One of Patañjali's innovations to the pre-existing body of yogic thought. It's aim is to reduce the *kleśas* directly as well as creating an enstatic state in the practitioner. It has three limbs:

tapas (ta-pas)

(See: II.1, II.32, II.43, IV.1)

Austerity and discipline. Practices that purify and refine the body and the senses.

svādhyāya (swahd-hee-yah-ya)

(See: II.1, II.32, II.44)

Self-study. Intense, self-directed study of the scriptures and, in modern interpretations, of the yogin's own body and consciousness.

īśvarapranidhana (eesh-wa-ra-pra-nid-ha-na)

(See: I.23, II.1, II.32, II.45)

An attitude of devotion towards *īśvara*, the supreme *puruṣa* that has never been tainted by *kleśa*, *saṃskāra* or manifestation in the material world.

2. *saṃyoga* (sang-yo-ga)

(See: II.17, II.23, II.25)

The tying together of observer with observed caused by *avidyā*, (misapprehension of one's own true nature) the primary *kleśa* that is the source of all the others. It is this that *Kriyā Yoga* aims to eliminate.

viveka (vi̲-ve̲-ka)

(See: II.26, II.28, III.52, III.54, IV.26, IV.29)

Discriminating discernment. The state of profound moment-to-moment awareness and discrimination necessary to separate observer from observed that will terminate *saṃyoga*.

Aṣṭāṅga Yoga

1. *aṣṭāṅga yoga* (ash-tah̲ng-ga yo̲-ga)

(See: II.28, II.29)

The eight limbed path of yoga. A comprehensive system that addresses the entirety of the practitioner's life, not merely his or her yogic practices. Although there is a progressive nature to the eight limbs, ultimately they are a wholistic system. The eight limbs are:

- Dealing with conduct and self-discipline:
  - *yama* - restraints
  - *niyama* - observances
- Dealing with harnessing the body, mind and senses:
  - *āsana* - posture
  - *prāṇāyāma* - restraint of the life force
  - *pratyāhāra* - withdrawal of the sense
- Dealing directly with the contents of consciousness
  - *dhāraṇā* - concentration
  - *dhyāna* - meditative absorption
  - *samādhi* - enstasy

2. *pratipakṣa bhāvana* (pra-ti-pa̲k-sha b-hah̲-va-na)

(See: II.33, II.34)

Cultivation of opposites. As a general palliative for unwholesome thoughts that will trigger deeper entrenchment of the *kleśas*, Patañjali offers us this as a practice to keep the mind clear by building up a storehouse of positive thoughts upon which to fall back in times of need.

3. *yama* (ya-ma)

(See: II.29, II.30)

The restraints. Patañjali refers to these as "The Great Vow of Yoga," or *mahāvratam*.

ahiṃsā (a-heeng-sah)

(See: II.30, II.35)

Non-harming. Grounding in this causes all enmity around the practitioner to be abandoned.

satya (sat-ya)

(See: II.30, II.36)

Truthfulness. Grounding in this causes all action and consequence to be grounded in truth for the practitioner.

asteya (as-tey-ya)

(See: II.30, II.37)

Non-stealing. Grounding in this provides abundance for the practitioner.

brahmacarya (bra-h-ma-char-ya)

(See: II.30, II.38)

Continence. Grounding in this brings vitality.

aparigraha (a-pa-ri-gra-ha)

(See: II.30, II.39)

Non-greed. Grounding in this brings knowledge of the subtle causes of the practitioner's birth.

4. niyama (nĭ-ya-ma)
(See: II.29, II.32)
The observances.

śauca (sha̱-oo-ca)
(See: II.32, II.40)
Purity of the body. With purity comes a sense of detachment from the body and disinterest in sullying it again with contact from others. Purity also brings serenity, gladness, single-pointed focus, mastery of the senses and the capacity for self-awareness.

saṃtosha (sa̱ng-to-sha)
(See: II.32, II.42)
Contentment, which brings the greatest joy.

tapas (ta̱-pas)
(See: II.1, II.32, II.43, IV.1)
Austerity and discipline. Practices that purify and refine the body and the senses.

svādhyāya (swahd-hee-ya̱h-ya)
(See: II.1, II.32, II.44)
Self-study. Intense, self-directed study of the scriptures and, in modern interpretations, or the yogin's own body and consciousness. Self-study establishes contact with the practitioner's *īṣṭadevatā*, or chosen deity.

īśvarapranidhana (ee̱sh-wa-ra-pra-nid-ha-na)
(See: I.23, II.1, II.32, II.45)
An attitude of devotion towards *īśvara*, the supreme *puruṣa* that has never been tainted by *kleśa*, *saṃskāra* or manifestation in the material world. This practice begins the perfection of enstasy.

5. *āsana* (ah-sa-na)

(See: II.29, II.46 to II.48)

Posture. Originally most likely referring to the posture of meditation, in recent centuries this has developed into the elaborate practices of *hatha yoga*. Patañjali tells us that one's posture should be effortlessly relaxed and infinitely expansive. If we can achieve this, we will be undisturbed by the buffeting of opposing forces such as heat and cold, or the pull of gravity from different directions.

6. *prāṇāyāma* (prah-nah-yah-ma)

(See: II.29, II.49 to II.53)

Restraint of the flow of the body's life force, the breath. This comes as a progression from correct posture. The breath can be conditioned along the lines of area of focus, or where the breath is happening in the body, duration of the breath itself and number of repetitions. Patañjali tells us that there is also a fourth aspect of breath that transcends all the others that can be conditioned. With this restraint, the practitioner's inner light can shine forth and the mind becomes fit for concentration.

7. *pratyāhāra* (pra-tyah-hah-ra)

(See: II.29, II.54)

Withdrawal of the senses. When the practitioner begins to detach him or herself from external objects and turns the senses inward. Not only does this have the effect of preparing the practitioner further for acts of single-pointed concentration, it also begins the subjugation of the senses to the practitioner's will.

8. *dhāraṇā* (d-hah-ra-nah)

(See: II.29, II.53, III.1)

Concentration. The binding of consciousness to one place. What we colloquially think of as "meditation" should really be thought of as concentration. It is a prerequisite for the next stage, meditative absorption, which will happen of its own accord or not, according to the level of restriction the practitioner is able to effect in his or her *vṛttis*.

9. dhyāna (d-hee-ah-na)

(See: I.39, II.11, II.29, III.2, IV.6)

Meditative absorption. Patañjali defines this as when all the *pratyayas* (notions) that fill the mind are directed towards the same place. Thus *dhyāna* is a deeper form of *dhāraṇā*, when the intention of single-pointed focus penetrates deeper down to the substratum beneath conscious thought.

pratyaya (pra-tya-ya)

(See: I.10, I.18, I.19, II.20, III.2, III.12, III.17, III.19, III.35, IV.27)

The cognitive representation of an object. The idea, the notion or the knowledge of that object. The mental model of an object. Everything that we know or perceive in the outside world has some form of representation in the *citta*.

10. samādhi (sam-ahd-hi)

(See: I.20, I.46, I.51, II.2, II.29, II.45, III.3, III.11, III.37, IV.1, IV.29)

Enstasy. When all conscious thought and all subconscious thought have merged in focus on the object of concentration, the object stands before the observer devoid of any connotations or connections at any level. The observer has reached a state beyond memory and identity. Then it becomes as if observer and observed are the same thing and the two merge. In this state the deep consciousness of the observer can begin to restructure and remodel itself along the lines of that perfect *puruṣa*, *īśvara*.

Samādhi and Kaivalya

1. samāpatti (sa-m<u>ah</u>-pat-ti)
(See: I.41, I.42, III.42)

The ability and tendency of *citta* to become like that which it observes. In the enstatic process, Patañjali uses the word to denoted particular stages in the inward progression of the practitioner.

savitarka samāpatti (n<u>i</u>r-vi-tar-ka sa-m<u>ah</u>-pat-ti)
(See: I.42)

Coincidence with thought. Observer and object have come together, but the practitioner's *citta* still exhibits conceptual knowledge based on language, the *vṛtti* known as *vikalpa*.

nirvitarka samāpatti (s<u>a</u>-vi-tar-ka sa-m<u>ah</u>-pat-ti)
(See: I.43)

Coincidence beyond thought. Once the deep memory *(smṛti)* has been purged of all *saṃskāras*, the observer can see the object without association or distortion.

savicāra samāpatti (nir-vi-ch<u>ah</u>-ra sa-m<u>ah</u>-pat-ti)
(See: I.44)

Coincidence with reflection. In the first two versions of *samāpatti*, the object of concentration is something gross outside of the practitioner's body. When the object is of a subtle nature that can lead the practitioner back to the source and there is still *vikalpa*, we have *savicāra samāpatti*.

nirvicāra samāpatti (sa-vi-ch<u>ah</u>-ra sa-m<u>ah</u>-pat-ti)
(See: I.44, I.47 to I.50)

Coincidence beyond reflection. With a subtle object and a purged *smṛti*, we have *nirvicāra samāpatti*. Patañjali also refers to this state as *vaiśāradya adhyātma* (va-ish-ah-ra-dya ad-hee-aht-ma), or "clarity of inner being." Peculiar to this state is an insight that reveals absolute truth and that lays down a new *saṃskāra* that obstructs all other *saṃskāras* from flaring up.

2. *sabīja samādhi* (sa-bee-ja sam-ahd-hi)

(See: I.46)

Enstasy with seed. The name Patañjali gives to the four *samāpattis*, given that in each there is some form of object around which the phenomenon coalesces.

samprajñāta samādhi (sang-praj-nyah-ta sam-ahd-hi)

(See: I.17)

Conscious enstasy. Another name given to the four *samāpattis*, by the many commentators to add their gloss on Patañjali in later centuries.

3. *nirbīja samādhi* (sa-bee-ja sam-ahd-hi)

(See: I.51)

Enstasy without seed. Occurs when the special restrictive *saṃskāra* that is laid down in *nirvicāra samāpatti* is also restrained. Also referred to by commentators as *asamprajñāta samādhi* (a-sang-praj-nyah-ta sam-ahd-hi) or enstasy beyond conscious thought. It is in this state that the three *pariṇāma* occur as the restructuring of the practitioner's consciousness develops.

nirodha pariṇāma (ni-rod-ha pa-ri-nah-ma)

(See: III.9 to III.10)

The "restriction transformation"; when the *saṃskāras* have been subjugated and new *saṃskāras* begin to emerge that promote further restriction.

samādhi pariṇāma (sa-m<u>ah</u>d-hi pa-ri-n<u>ah</u>-ma)
(See: III.11)

The "integration transformation"; when the outward dissipation of *citta* begins to dwindle and a consistent state of single-pointed focus emerges.

ekāgratā pariṇāma (ey-k<u>ah</u>-gra-t<u>ah</u> pa-ri-n<u>ah</u>-ma)
(See: III.12)

The "single-pointedness transformation"; when the quieting and the dissipating contents of *citta* become balanced.

4. saṃyama (s<u>ang</u>-ya-ma)
(See: III.4, III.16, III.17, III.21, III.22, III.26, III.35, III.41, III.42, III.44, III.47, III.52)

Constraint. The term for bringing to bear all three of the final limbs of *aṣṭāṅga yoga* — *dhāraṇā, dhyāna, samādhi* — on a particular object. Patañjali lists many powers, or *vibhūti* (vib-h<u>oo</u>-ti), which can be acquired by the yogin as result of this practice.

5. dharma-megha-samādhi (d-h<u>a</u>r-ma m<u>e</u>g-ha sam-<u>ah</u>d-hi)
(See: IV.29)

Cloud of Virtue. The penultimate stage prior to complete emancipation. Results from the practitioner being able to remain dispassionate and discriminating in the state of *nirbīja samādhi* after *ekāgratā-pariṇāma*, the single-pointedness transformation.

6. kaivalya (k<u>ai</u>-val-ya)
(See: II.25, III.50, III.55, IV.26, IV.34)

Aloneness. Emancipated freedom. The final stage, in which *citta* has become completely *sattvic*, the *guṇas* have flowed back to the source and the ultimate purpose of *prakṛti* has been fulfilled.

Sanskrit Pronunciation Guide

Vowels

a	short, sounds like b*u*t
ā	long, sounds like *a*rm
i	short, sounds like b*i*t
ī	long, sounds like s*ee*
u	short, sounds like f*oo*t
ū	long, sounds like f*oo*d
e	sounds like pl*ay*
o	sounds like h*o*pe
ṛ	a lightly sounded "r" as in rolling the "r" in p*r*etty
ai, ay	sound like r*i*de
au	sounds like n*ow*

Consonants

ka, kha, ga, gha, ṅa	gutturals (sounded in the back of the throat)
ca, cha, ja, jha, ña	palatals (sounded on the soft palate)
ṭa, ṭha, ḍa, ṭha, ṇa	cerebrals (sounded behind the teeth)
ta, tha, da, dha, na	dentals (sounded on the teeth)
pa, pha, ba, bha, ma	labials (sounded on the lips)
s	as in *s*ent
ś, ṣ	as in *sh*out
ñ	as in ca*ny*on
c, j	always soft, as in *ch*ill, *j*oy
h, r	always sounded, as in up*h*ill, ac*r*id
ḥ	*visarga* – the preceding vowel is lightly repeated
ṃ	*anusvāra* – as in sa*ng*

Bibliography

Arya, P. U. (1986) *Yoga-Sutras of Patañjali with the Exposition of Vyasa: A Translation and Commentary, Volume I.* Himalayan International Institute, Honesdale, PA.

Desikachar, T. K. V. (1995) *The Heart of Yoga: Developing a Personal Practice.* Inner Traditions International, Rochester, VT.

Feuerstein, G. (1989 [1979]) *The Yoga-Sutra of Patañjali: A New Translation and Commentary.* Inner Traditions International, Rochester, VT.

— (1996) *The Philosophy of Classical Yoga.* Inner Traditions International, Rochester, VT.

— (1997) *The Shambhala Encyclopedia of Yoga.* Shambhala Publications, Inc., Boston, MA.

— (1998) *The Yoga Tradition.* Hohm Press, Prescott, AZ.

Hartranft, C. (2003) *The Yoga-Sutra of Patañjali: A New Translation with Commentary.* Shambhala Classics, Boston, MA.

Iyengar, B. K. S. (1979 [1966]) *Light on Yoga: Yoga Dipika.* Inner Traditions Schocken Books, New York, NY.

— (1993) *Light on the Yoga Sutras of Patañjali: Patañjala Yoga Pradipika.* Aquarian/Thorsons, San Francisco, CA.

Sri Swami Satchidananda. (1990 [1987]) *The Yoga Sutras of Patañjali: A New Translation and Commentary.* Integral Yoga Publications, Yogaville, VA.

About the Author

Witold Fitz-Simon was born in London, England in 1967. After growing up in England and Brazil, Witold moved to the United States in 1985 to study film at NYU's Tisch School of the Arts where he received an Honours B.F.A. He began to study yoga and meditation as an antidote to a stressful career in the entertainment industry with yoga teacher and choreographer Colleen Winney. He followed that with several years of study at the world-renowned Jivamukti Yoga Center, studying primarily with Katchie Ananda Gaard, immersing himself in their physically intense and devotional style of vinyasa.

After a yoga-related injury in 1995, Witold retreated from the classroom to practice on his own with B.K.S. Iyengar's seminal book, "Light on Yoga." A year of solitary practice led him to the Iyengar Yoga Institute of New York, where he felt an immediate connection to Mr. Iyengar's way of working. In 2000, Fitz-Simon embraced the yoga lifestyle and began teaching yoga full time after extensive training at the Iyengar Institute under Robin Janis and at the "Yogaville" Integral Yoga Ashram in Virginia. There he was fortunate enough to hear the late, world-renowned Swami Satchidananda teach on several occasions, and was awarded the Sanskrit name *Shankara*, "the bliss-maker." He is a registered yoga instructor and teacher-trainer with Yoga Alliance.

Witold continues to teach and write about yoga full-time in the New York area. He is author of the "Yoga Practice Journal," also published by Dedo Press. For information about his classes, visit www.wyoga.com, and to read more of his writing, visit www.yogaartandscience.com. He can be reached at witold@wyoga.com

CPSIA information can be obtained at www.ICGtesting.com
Printed in the USA
BVOW071756030213

312283BV00001B/3/A

9 780977 173310